DATE DUE			

SPORTS
FOR THE
HANDICAPPED

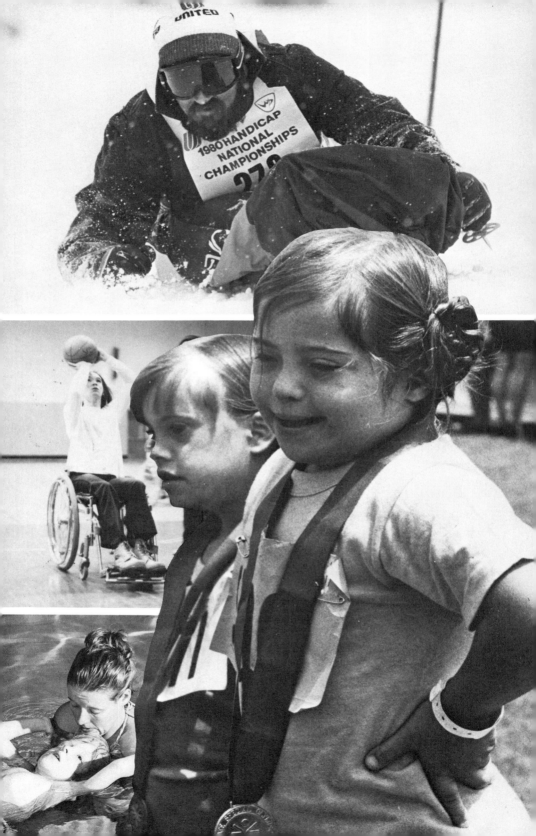

SPORTS
FOR THE
HANDICAPPED

By ANNE ALLEN

WALKER AND COMPANY ☀ New York, New York

For George, Billy, and Sammy

796.0196
ALSs
124139
Mar.1983

Library of Congress Cataloging in Publication Data

Allen, Anne.
  Sports for the handicapped.

  1. Sports for the physically handicapped.
I. Title.
GV709.3.A44   796'.01'96   81-50738
ISBN 0-8027-6436-3   AACR2
ISBN 0-8027-6437-1 (lib. bdg.)

All the characters and events portrayed in this story are fictitious.

First published in the United States of America in 1981 by the Walker Publishing Company, Inc.

Published simultaneously in Canada by John Wiley & Sons Canada Limited, Rexford, Ontario

ISBN: 0-8027-6436-3 (Trade)
        0-8027-6437-1 (Reinforced)

Library of Congress Catalog Card Number: 81-50739

Book designed by Lena Fong Hor

Printed in the United States of America

10 9 8 7 6 5 4 3 2 1

Contents

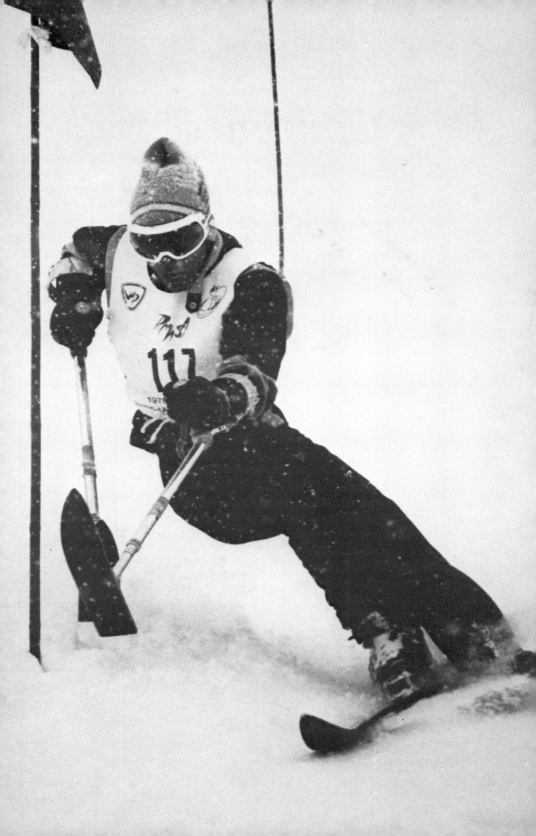

Introduction

Once there was no such thing as sports for disabled people, but after World War II, the many young men who came out of the conflict with limited physical abilities due to injuries demanded to participate in some form of sports. The revolution in athletics for the disabled began with the efforts of the famed British physician, Dr. Ludwig Guttman, to reintegrate these young men into the everyday lives of their communities. He founded the Spinal Injury Center in Stoke Mandeville, England, and in 1948 organized the first athletic contest for handicapped athletes.

Today, physically-limited athletes participate in every sport—including hang gliding and sky diving. The disabled athletes compete not only with each other, but more and more, they are competing in standard athletic events against the able-bodied. In the 1980 Boston Marathon, for instance, four contestants in wheelchairs crossed the line ahead of able-bodied winner Bill Rodgers.

A young Cambodian named Ri Robert Armstrong had his left leg amputated below the knee following an injury in the Vietnam War. Adopted by an American family, he learned three-track skiing at Winter Park, Colorado. He captured the national junior three-track championship and later went on to win third place, silver medalist in the men's division. While doing this, Ri went out for basketball, not with a team for the disabled, but with a regular able-bodied team in

Robert Armstrong, 1981 Third Place, Silver Medalist. Men's National Handicap Three-Track Ski Championships at Winter Park, Colorado.

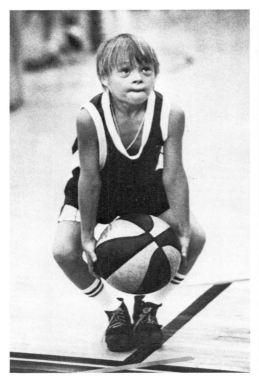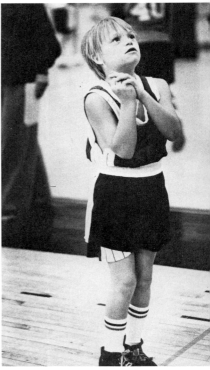

the Denver city league. The only physically-limited member of the team, Ri became captain. He led the team to the Denver city-wide championship for six straight years.

The man who taught Ri to ski is Hal O'Leary. For ten years, he has been director of the skiing program for the handicapped at Winter Park and in that time, he has seen many remarkable performances like Ri's.

Hal says that if you can stand he can teach you to ski. Under Hal's instruction an eight-year-old boy with prostheses on both legs and both arms learned to ski. And if you can't stand, Hal has a ski-sled in which you can still slam down a mountain to experience the wonderful sensation of having your cheeks whipped by the cold, clear air, while hearing the marvelous, shussing sound of skis racing over powdered snow.

"The physically-limited feel society is pressing them to prove themselves," Hal explains. "More and more, they are driven to achieve performances in athletics none of us would have thought

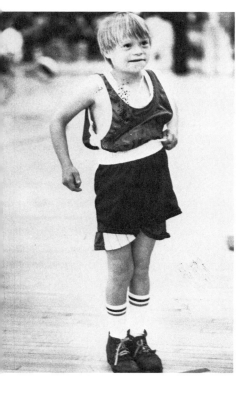

Whether it lands in the basket . . . or not . . . doesn't matter . . . the idea is to have fun. *Courtesy Special Olympics*

possible twenty, or even ten years ago."

For the 35 million physically-limited people in the United States, athletics bring the same rewards sports do for the able-bodied—a healthier body, an improved mental outlook, and a widened social life. In addition, the disabled athletes get something extra—the satisfaction of stretching themselves farther than they thought they could, the indescribable joy of crossing the finish line ahead of someone else.

Winning, however, is not what athletics for the disabled is all about. The most important thing is participation, and that winners serve as models to show others what can be achieved despite physical or mental limitations.

For the mentally retarded one of the best known sports programs is the Special Olympics. The Joseph P. Kennedy Foundation began the Special Olympics in 1968 and since then, more than two million mentally retarded people have participated in both national and international events.

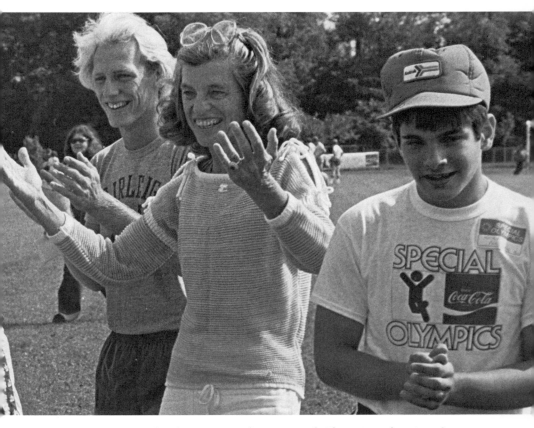

Eunice Kennedy Shriver, President, Special Olympics, cheering the team.
Courtesy Special Olympics

"More than single victories or trophies," said Mrs. Eunice Kennedy Shriver, President of the Special Olympics, "our greatest respect and admiration go to all who try, who make a gallant effort, who stay in the race, no matter where they finish."

There are Special Olympics programs throughout the country. They offer sixteen sports to suit everyone's liking, with basketball and soccer the most popular. To participate, mentally retarded persons need only to have passed their eighth birthday. There is no upper age limit.

It has now been proved that every person of limited ability can participate in some sport. For every sport in which the physically-limited participate, there is now an organization. In almost every city in the nation there is now a sports program for the handi-capped. To find one, start by checking the Y's, the Red Cross, and the 4-H Clubs. There is a resource list of organizations at the back of this book.

A word of caution: your watchword must always be safety first. Just as with able-bodied athletes, you can injure yourself by working too hard, going too fast, or by not having the proper in-struction in how to do it right. Talk to your doctor and get his per-mission before you start. Find an instructor who has had training in adaptive physical education.

Remember that athletics for the physically-limited are *not* intended to be therapeutic only. You shouldn't work at them grimly. The main idea is to have fun. If you achieve that, then other benefits will follow.

There is a much wider world out there for disabled people than there used to be. The attitude of the able-bodied—and the disabled themselves—toward what disabled people are capable of has been changing rapidly.

This changing attitude is well illustrated by the experience of the world-famous violinist, Itzak Perlman. After a concert the news-paper headline the next day would read "Disabled violinist plays brilliantly." Perlman used to grit his teeth at the attitude these reports indicated. For, as he explained, his disability affected only his legs, and legs aren't used in playing the violin. Nowadays the re-views hardly ever refer to his disability. If it is mentioned at all, it appears near the end of the review.

What this book tries to show is that neither the form of your dis-ability nor your age is any barrier. There is a sport for you and specially trained experts are available to help you.

So, go and enjoy!

Anne Allen
April 1981

11

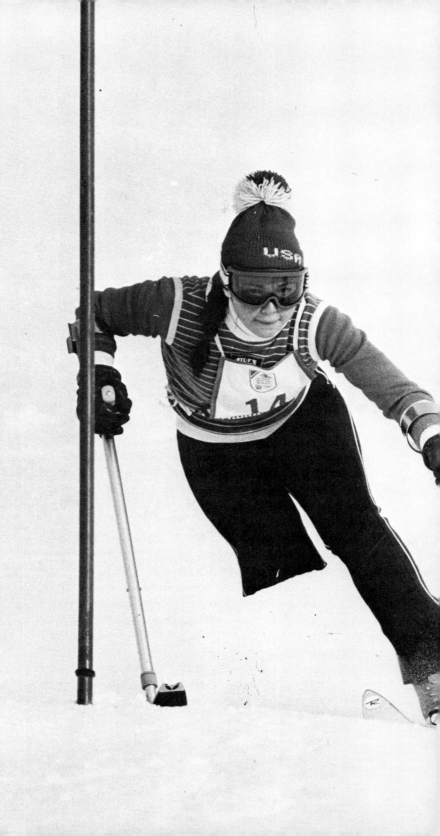

Skiing

On a cold day, Diana Golden was running through the woods near her home. She was in the 7th grade, 12 years old, and she and her friend had just built a fort. Now she was running as fast as she could, her long, dark, braided hair flying around her face, as she tried to beat her best friend out of the woods into the meadow. Laughing, she shouted, "Come on, I'll race you home."

But then Diana fell. Her right leg simply stopped working. She sprawled on the cold ground with the dirt and fallen leaves.

Catching up, Diana's friend asked, "Are you o.k.?"

"I'm all right, just a tumble." Laughing, Diana brushed herself off and quickly got up.

She tried to walk, but she couldn't. She started to limp, thinking she had simply bruised her leg.

When the limping persisted for several days her parents took her to the doctor. Two weeks went by and she continued to limp and now Diana was in terrible pain, almost all the time.

Two months later, a doctor discovered what was wrong with Diana. She had cancer. They removed her right leg above the knee.

Five years after the operation, in the spring of 1980, Diana, now age 17, wearing Number 14 on her ski jacket, zoomed out of the starting gate at the Winter Handicap Olympics in Geilo, Norway. Diana was an official member of the American Ski Team, representing her country and showing the world what a handicapped skier

Diana Golden, considered one of the better three-track skiers in the U.S., showing what she can do.

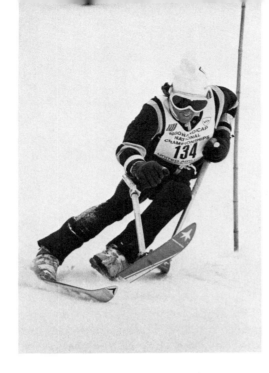

David Jamison, 1981 Men's National Handicap Three-track Ski Champion. *Photo by Bruce Benedict, Winter Park*

can do. The races are held every four years, and the team is competitively chosen and represents the best handicapped ski athletes in the U.S.

She participated in the giant slalom and the slalom. Though she didn't win, she sometimes hit 60 mph on the hills. Her spirit, however, demonstrated something far more important than winning—courage.

The powerful will-to-win attitude of most competitive athletes is part of Diana's character. But before flying off to Norway, her father taught her a very important lesson about winning and losing.

"I love to win, but I love the skiing itself more than winning. I know that sometimes I will get caught up in the win thing and then it's no fun. The point is to get as good as you can, and if as good as you can isn't going to win, well then, you keep trying, but you just enjoy yourself while you are at it.

"So many kids feel they have to win for their parents. But, my Dad, he's really neat in the way he talks to me. He said, 'Do you think it makes any difference to me if you win or lose?' I said, No.

"'You are absolutely wrong,' he told me. 'I'd love it if you win. I would tell the whole world. But you're you to me—and win or lose, I'm going to love you anyway. It's not going to be the end of my world if you lose. So, I don't want you to feel that you have to win for me.'

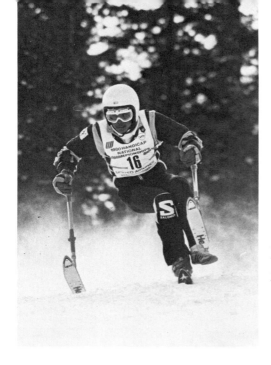

A three-track skier whose fast turn leaves a cloud of snow behind him. *Photo by Bruce Benedict, Winter Park*

"When I came back from Norway, I felt awful because I didn't win. But I knew it wasn't going to matter to my parents. They were going to be glad I had a good time in Norway."

To train for the Norway races required grit and determination on Diana's part. But she modestly labels that determination 'stubbornness' and says it sometimes gets in her way.

"I was convinced that skiing with poles was the best way—one ski and regular poles. Last year when I was on the ski team, I skied with regular ski poles.

"At the Nationals in Colorado, I skied with regular poles, but I got too excited and went overboard. I tried to go faster when everybody told me to go slower, because I had the race won, if I had only finished it."

Amputees have a choice of skiing either with two skis, wearing one ski on their artificial leg, or on only one ski. If they use two skis, they use regular ski poles like everybody else. But if they use only one ski, it is better for them to use outriggers in place of regular ski poles. Instead of the sharp tip and the round metal piece at the bottom of regular ski poles, the outriggers have little skis on the bottom. When you ski with outriggers, you leave behind a track showing three ski trails. So this way of skiing is called "three-track" skiing. Diana prefers to ski three-track.

Diana owns two artificial legs. One she calls a "leg-leg." It has a foot and a knee joint and she wears it most of the time. When she goes skiing, however, she prefers to use her other one. It's a peg-leg, like the one old Long John Silver wore. It's made of aluminum, is very light, and it is made in two pieces. The bottom part snaps on or off the socket section in a second or two. Diana prefers to ski with one ski, but at the bottom of the hill she needs an artificial leg for walking around and getting to the lift or to the restaurant. She prefers the peg-leg for this, because she can unsnap it so quickly and leave it at the bottom of the hill next to the lift.

Once someone threw out her peg-leg, thinking it was a stray piece of metal someone had left behind. But the ski team helped Diana search for it. They found it in the trash bin.

"One of the nice things about wearing the socket and peg-leg is that it protects your stump," Diana explained. "I have almost stopped wearing the peg for skiing because I had a bad habit of keeping my stump out to the side for balance. It's better if you keep it tucked in tight, your two legs together. If you keep your stump out, you don't make your turns as precise. Everything counts, your body angle and everything.

"In Norway, I had to ski with outriggers because that is what the rules say. I also finally learned outriggers are better for me than regular poles, because after I fall I can get going again more easily with outriggers."

Diana spent the summer of 1980 living and working with a young Amish-Mennonite farm family in Pennsylvania. She did her share of the farm chores and helped Mary Ellen, the farmer's wife, with the cooking and sometimes cared for their two-year-old son. Diana's energy level impressed the hard-working farm couple.

Her left leg showed all the signs of farm living, mosquito bites, poison ivy, briar scratches and suntan. But about her right leg she said, "One good thing about having my leg-leg is that it doesn't get poison ivy or bites. All I have to do is wash it.

"But in the afternoon when I take a nap, it sure feels good to take it off. I might take a nap and leave it on sometimes, but I don't particularly like to, it isn't comfortable. It's like sleeping with ski boots on. When you come in from skiing, you just love to take your heavy ski boots off and relax your feet. It's the same with an artificial leg. It just feels so good to take it off and relax a little bit from it."

Today Diana is considered one of the better three-track women skiers in the United States. At times her performance has been better than two-legged skiers. But it wasn't always that way.

"I was the original klutz," she laughed. "In the 5th grade, we moved from one city to another. I was the new kid and in the 5th, 6th, and pretty much in the 7th grades, the other kids picked on me and I was always in tears. Then after I lost my leg, things changed a lot. I learned that the kids weren't going to say anything to me. I could be the way I wanted to be. So that gave me new self-confidence.

"I wanted to join the ski-team in school. I was on the swim team for a little bit, then it got in the way of training for skiing, so I dropped swimming. Before I lost my leg, I had skied, but never competitively.

"To develop my body for tough competitive skiing, I started taking gym classes and gymnastics. I also took Yoga and outward-bound-type classes."

When the ski team jogged, Diana made up her own exercise which she calls 'crutching' or 'crogging.'

"Have you ever seen anyone hop between crutches? I go crutch-hop-crutch-hop, it's kind of like jogging.

"I couldn't do one single push-up when I started on the ski team. By the time I finished the ski season, I could do 19 push-ups in one minute. Right now, I can do 25 without stopping.

"At first when I exercised with the ski team, I couldn't do some of the exercises. For instance, they would stand on one leg and then lift another. Having just one leg, I couldn't do that. But then I figured out a way to do the exercise sitting on the floor.

"I was never an athletic person before I lost my leg. That's just the way it was. When kids were choosing sides for a game, the klutz is always chosen last and that was me. Losing my leg taught me that you can train your body. It is not all a matter of having natural athletic ability. If you put in the effort, you can train yourself.

"Some kids say to me, 'Well, I can't do even one push-up.' And I say, you've never worked at doing push-ups long enough, that's why. It's a matter of discipline."

Some people think that amputees must be sad and gloomy because a part of their body is missing. But that isn't so with Diana. She has a sunny personality—and a good sense of humor concerning her missing leg.

"When I am on my crutches, some of my friends call me 'tripod,'" she giggled. "I don't mind because I know it is said with love and caring. When I wear my peg-leg, other friends call me 'peg-gy.'"

Diana tries to put people at ease about her artificial leg. She makes it easy for them to ask questions or to help her.

"That's part of my job, or of any person who is handicapped. If they make others feel awkward around them, that is partially their fault. People will automatically feel awkward at first, but if you lead them, they'll get over it."

Diana always extends a helping hand to others who are newly handicapped, who often are confused and don't know where to turn for help. Diana will comfort and advise a new friend who has been recently handicapped, drawing on her own experience as a disabled person.

"There was a girl who wanted to learn horseback riding and she really didn't know what to do," Diana recalled. "Well, I explained what she needed and told her where she could have a special socket made up so she could ride a horse."

Diana explained that riders who have two good legs keep their balance by gripping the horse with their lower legs and with their thighs, something a person with only one leg cannot do. Amputees ride by means of a leather socket that is attached to the saddle. They place a specially-designed plastic socket over their stump and fit the lower end into the leather socket. This arrangement permits them to keep their balance and avoid falling off as they lean with the horse as it turns.

Diana's Pointers For the Handicapped

"If you can't find someone in your neighborhood who has the same kind of disability as you do, then go to the library and check it out.

"You have to take the initiative and not be afraid to search for help. Like getting the proper prosthesis—my artificial leg-leg—I really had to search to find the man I use now. If I go into the workshop where they make artificial legs with a problem and I think it is something they can't take care of, my Mom will say, 'Well, ask him Diana?' Finally, I ask him and he takes care of it. He does a good job and he cares so much.

"Don't be afraid of your prosthesis. The first year in high school, I would go to school without my prosthesis. I was too embarrassed. In junior year when I started ski team, I started to get used to it. I used to wear a long stocking all the time to cover it. Then when I got my peg-leg, I started to wear it to school because it was so light. At

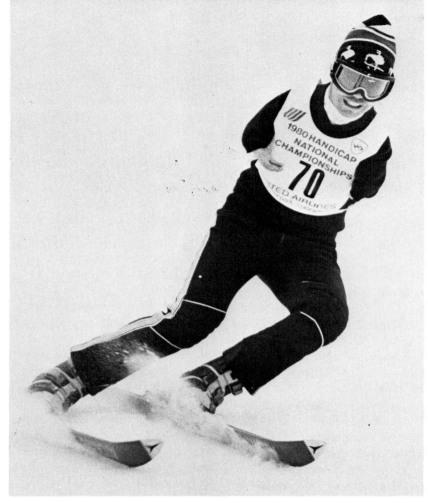

A skier without arms demonstrating an expert manuever. *Photo by Bruce Benedict, Winter Park*

first, I would always wear slacks because I was embarrassed. Then one day I said to a school friend, do you think I could wear a skirt? She replied, 'Yes! It's a beautiful shiny leg.'

"During gym classes, while I was training hard for Norway, I would take off my leg-leg and a couple of times during the day, I would stick it in the locker. The girls beside me looked a little startled at first, but then it didn't matter. They would go by my reaction, if it didn't bother me, why should it bother them.

"Don't ever say 'I can't.' Accept yourself as a human being. Don't consider yourself less because you don't have all your senses—you are blind or deaf—or because you are missing a part of your body. Don't stop. Maybe you are not able to do something now, but maybe you will be able to do it later. Be happy with where you are and where you are going.

"Don't be afraid to fall. You'll learn a lot. If a kid falls, people run over and say, 'Can I pick you up?' Well, when you do that you are telling the kid he is helpless. If you are always there to pick up that child, then he will never learn to pick himself up.

"I am not a handicapped person. I know my right leg is gone, but I don't consider myself handicapped. I can get handicapped license plates—and although it would be nice for my parents to have them, so they can park anywhere—I'm not going to get them now because that would be saying I am handicapped.

"For every physical disability there is a solution."

The Nation's Best Ski Instruction for the Handicapped

A great deal of credit for solving the problems of the handicapped can go to Hal O'Leary, who ten years ago pioneered the ski program at Winter Park, Colorado, which is close to Denver. Today Winter Park has more than 240 instructors.

More than 500 physically-limited children and adults take ski classes each week of the season. During the past ten years, 5,000 children and adults have learned to ski at Winter Park. Each trainee is given one-to-one instruction. If special equipment is necessary, it is tailored to fit the need.

Participants in the ski program include those who are blind, deaf, mentally retarded, paraplegics, those who have cerebral palsy, post-polio, multiple sclerosis, congenital defects, and spina bifida.

Before entering the ski program at Winter Park, the student is screened to determine the nature of the handicap. Is one leg shorter than the other? Are both legs involved? The ski equipment is then adapted to fit the need. Those with limited use of their arms and legs ski three-track or four-track. Many of the three-track instructors at Winter Park are themselves amputees.

Four-track skiing is used by people who have limited use of both legs. They use two skis and two outriggers.

Those who have experienced loss of muscle tone because of muscular dystrophy or spina bifida, for example, are taught to use a ski bra. It's a metal device that links both skis at the tips. It enables the skier to maintain a parallel position and do a snowplow.

A ski sled for paraplegics is a new device now being used at

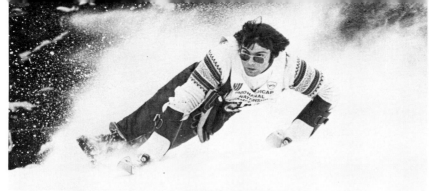

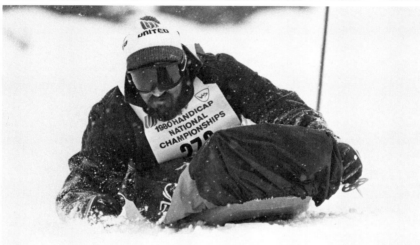

(Above) Rene Kirby, who learned to ski on his hands. *Photo by Bruce Benedict. (Below)* A ski sled for paraplegics. Sometimes called by the Norwegian name, *pulk,* or an arroya, it is a one-man toboggan propelled with the aid of ice poles called stickers. *Photo by Bruce Benedict*

Winter Park. Sometimes called by the Norwegian name, *pulk,* it is a one-man toboggan which is propelled with the aid of ice poles called stickers. It is used for downhill skiing and fits onto conventional chairlifts.

At Winter Park, the big event of the year is the week-long Handicapped National Championships. More than 200 participants ranging in age from 7 to 70 from all over the country competed last Spring. The skiers were classified according to age and disability. To the spectators who watched them, they represented courage and dedication.

Says Hal O'Leary: "The true satisfaction comes from the realization that, as an individual, on a one-to-one basis with himself, this person has accomplished something that he perhaps never dreamed that he could do. He is skiing."

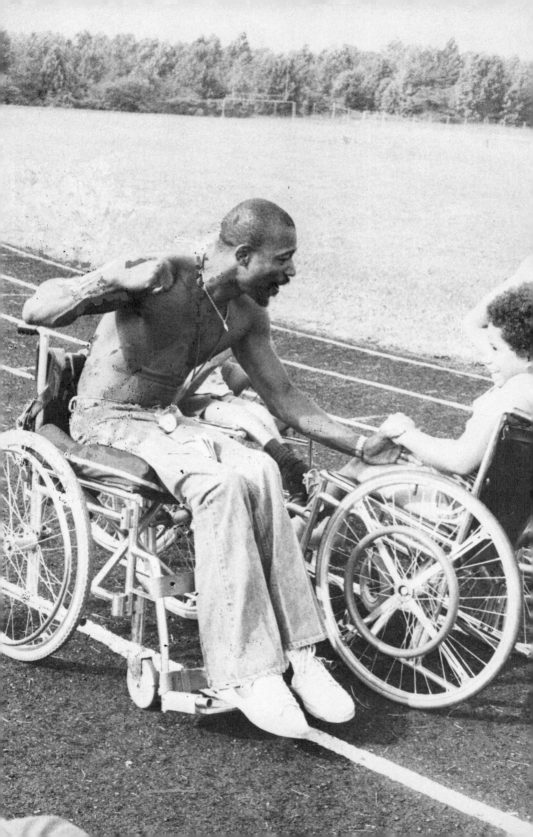

Wheelchair Basketball

When Bill Greene was 16, he was accidentally shot. He was paralyzed from the waist down and was in despair, thinking his life was over. He felt he might as well be dead. For six years he did little but wallow in self-pity.

Then he discovered wheelchair basketball. He fell in love with the game and it has radically changed his life, not only physically, but emotionally and spiritually as well.

Now an expert at wheelchair sports, Bill is devoting his life to sharing his abilities and enthusiasm with other paraplegics who need to be shown that they can do a great deal more than they believe—and help improve their lives—by participating in organized sports. He is a counselor at a school for handicapped children. Street-wise, but possessed of charm and grace, along with a powerful drive to help, Bill has all the tools needed to motivate handicapped youngsters to try harder and to succeed.

Ten years ago, with his wife Brenda, who is able-bodied, Bill started *New Life, Inc.,* a non-profit sports program to train those in wheelchairs to become competitive athletes. Based in the nation's capital, the program includes basketball, track and field events and swimming.

Brenda is an elementary school teacher. After school hours, she devotes all her time to *New Life.* She takes care of all the scheduling, transportation, and coordinating. Bill is the coach/trainer.

During the summer, the younger children learn how to use their wheelchairs in sports. During the fall and winter, the *New Life* basketball team, the *Capital Smokers,* competes in a 12-game conference schedule, plus an additional 12-game schedule with top-ranked teams around the country. Every November, *New Life* spon-

Bill Greene, director and co-founder of New Life, Inc., gives Charla Ramsey a pep talk. *Photo courtesy Brenda Greene*

sors a two-day wheelchair invitational basketball tournament. Also during the fall and winter, a swimming program operates in tandem with the basketball program. In the spring, the program concentrates on track and field events.

Sixty athletes of both sexes, some as young as eight years old, participate. One of them, Sylvester Fiers, 21, won five first-place medals at the 1980 Olympics for the Disabled in Arnhem, Holland. Sylvester started training with Bill when he was 13 years old. It took Bill only five years to turn him into an Olympic contender.

Bill says there are no scientific studies that *prove* organized sports are beneficial for people in wheelchairs. But Bill knows from practical experience that sports are good for paraplegics—in exactly the same way that sports are good for the able-bodied.

"The benefits, physically, are just outstanding," he says. "The mental benefits come from the physical benefits because you feel better. Wheelchair sports are not gentle, panty-waist games. They are played fast and hard and to compete, you have to get into shape and stay in shape. Half of playing wheelchair basketball, for instance, is the ability to push the chair—push it fast, be able to accelerate, stop on a dime, and turn quickly. And you have to do all this with one hand, because you have to dribble the ball and shoot with the other."

To train for the competitive season, Bill, who is the playing coach, brings his basketball team, the *Capital Smokers,* together right after Labor Day. The training schedule is tough, four days a week. They meet at a quarter-mile track. Each player starts by doing eight laps while dribbling the ball. These first laps are easy. Bill lets each player do them at his own speed. Each must stay within his lane, which is good training in how to steer their chairs accurately. After the eight laps, the team does fast dribbling quarters, racing each other. Next comes three fast hundreds, then three fast fifties.

"Then we do sprints up a steep ramp for five minutes. After that we practice on the court for an hour and a half," explained Bill.

Team members do a lot of grousing about the tough practice. Bill ignores the complaints because he knows—and he knows every one of his athletes knows—that they must build strength, endurance, and accuracy. Since wheelchair athletes are prone to hand blisters, they also need lots of practice to toughen their hands. "Good conditioning also helps us to avoid injuries on the court," Bill explains.

The physically demanding training schedule for the *Capital Smokers* is based on Bill's own experience at Wichita State Uni-

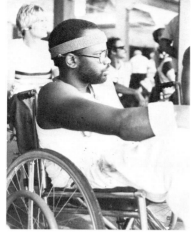

Sylvester Fiers watching his New Life teammates. *Photo courtesy Brenda Greene*

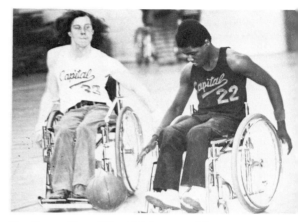

Ray Joers, *(l)* and David Johnson of the Capital Smokers basketball team during a practice session. *Photo courtesy Brenda Greene*

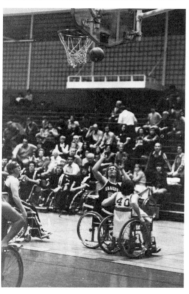

A University of Illinois Gizz Kid shoots for the basket. *Photo by Dr. Frank Maglione, Rehabilitation Education Center, University of Illinois*

versity and on expert advice. Wheelchair basketball coach Ed Owens, of the University of Kentucky, nationally recognized as an authority on the sport, visits *New Life* twice a year to put on demonstration clinics. Another expert, Dr. Julian Stein, of the American Alliance of Health, Physical Education, Recreation, and Dance, also advises Bill.

Watching the *Capital Smokers* play the University of Illinois' wheelchair basketball team, the *Gizz Kids,* a spectator described what she saw as "the closest thing to disco dancing on wheels." The players whirl and spin their chairs with great dexterity. There is nothing meek about the game. Sometimes players fall out of their chairs. Some can scramble unaided back onto their seats. For

25

others, an able-bodied bystander quickly lends a hand. The agility of the wheelchair players with their hands, arms, and upper torsos is dazzling. From their sitting position, they easily shoot baskets, loop the ball in any direction to teammates, feint and fake shots. The play is fast and accurate. There is no clumsiness. As in able-bodied basketball, players keep up a chatter: "Take your time . . . I've got 34 . . . Block him . . . Come on, John . . . Over here, Mike . . . Good shot, Sharon!" Players spin about the court so fast and with such aggressive determination that inexperienced spectators often fear that the chairs and players will end up as a mess of mangled steel and flesh. It never happens. Players can stop their chairs on a dime. dime."

The rules of wheelchair basketball have been kept as close as possible to those of the able-bodied game. Court size and basket height are the same. A major difference is that the chair is considered part of the person, so that roughness against the chair is considered roughness against the player in it. As in able-bodied basketball, there is a penalty for unnecessary roughness.

There are some minor differences in the rules. In the able-bodied game, if you dribble and stop, you are not allowed to dribble again. In the wheelchair game you can dribble, stop, and dribble again. In the wheelchair game, players must remain seated. If they lift their hips off the chair, it is considered a physical-advantage foul. In the able-bodied game, a player is allowed only three seconds in the free-throw lane. A wheelchair player has five seconds.

Some players use special basketball chairs. They are lighter, so they are easier to push, and they don't have arms, which allows occupants greater freedom of movement with their upper body.

Bill believes the most important function of wheelchair sports is to raise a player's self-esteem. Bill constantly works against something he calls "negative thinking."

"Many youngsters who join *New Life* start out discouraged," he explains. "They are beaten, down and out, feeling they can't do a thing. A lot of that attitude is the fault of able-bodied relatives and

(Top) University of Illinois Gizz Kids mixing it up with the Chicago University basketball team. In the heat of the game, players often slip from their chairs, but are seldom hurt. *Photo by Dr. Frank Maglione. (Middle)* A University of Illinois Gizz Kid goes after the ball. *Photo by Emiko Miyasaka. (Bottom)* Brad Hedrick, University of Illinois Gizz Kid, tries to keep his balance. *Photo by Emiko Miyasaka*

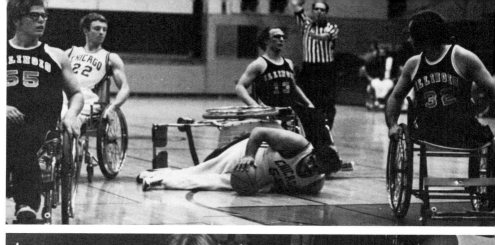

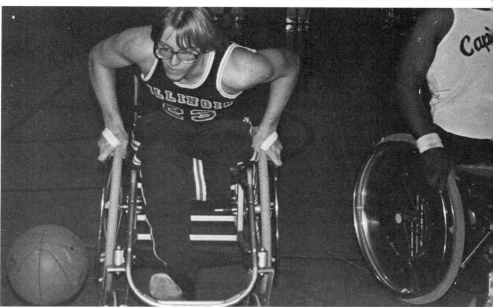

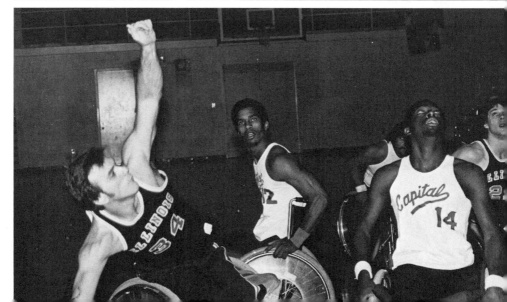

friends who do not expect much from the handicapped. As a result, the disabled don't expect much of themselves. That attitude is harmful. It's a terrible psychological trap."

Bill ought to know. For years he had such an attitude. He thought he was a loser.

At 16, Bill was running around with some tough company. He had been thrown out of two high schools and was about to repeat the 10th grade for the third time. He found school to be boring. When he did go, it was to hang around the playground. One day two of Bill's friends got into a fight. He tried to break it up. A pistol went off, accidentally shooting Bill. The bullet lodged in his spinal cord and paralyzed his legs.

"I got shot on my mother's birthday," he recalled, "which I thought was a terrible birthday present."

He spent the next 22 months in the hospital. His parents stuck by him. Without their courage and support, Bill doubts he could have made the transition from an active, able-bodied youngster to a paraplegic without losing his mind. "After I was hurt there never was a time that my parents weren't supportive of what I was doing. That meant a great deal to me."

Bill's parents made sure he continued his education while he was in the hospital and with the help of a tutor, he completed high school. That was as far as Bill wanted to go. Angry and feeling sorry for himself, Bill felt he was just too dumb to go any further. But he hadn't reckoned with his father, who kept urging Bill to think of college. Every time the subject was raised, Bill said no. His father persisted, never letting go of the idea. Finally, only to get his father off his back, Bill agreed to try college, never believing he would ever get there.

"While I agreed with my father, I was still saying in my heart, 'I really can't do this.' I think it's very important for everybody to understand that many disabled people have that attitude, not only about academics, but about all of life."

Bill enrolled at Wichita State University in Emporia, Kansas. It is a barrier-free school where all the handicapped students live on the first floor of the dormitory. Not long after, the University of Illinois, which is considered the national center of wheelchair sports, gave a wheelchair basketball exhibition game at Wichita State. That game was the turning point for Bill.

"I guess I was 22 years old at the time. You can imagine my anger when I found out that there were things like this going on and I

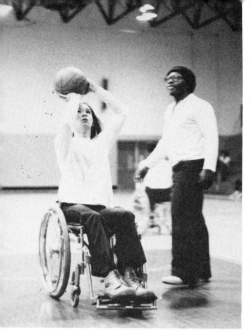

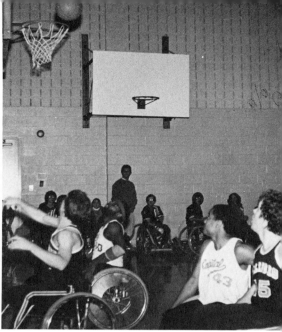

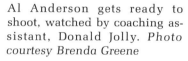

Al Anderson gets ready to
shoot, watched by coaching assistant, Donald Jolly. *Photo
courtesy Brenda Greene*

A Gizz Kid dunks the ball.
Photo by Emiko Miyasaka

didn't know about them. Wheelchair sports would have been terrific
motivation for me when I was 16 years old. I could have directed a
lot of my hostilities about being disabled into positive channels and
got rid of them. I felt I had wasted six years."

Another milestone in Bill's life was passed later in Kansas. Two
days after receiving his Master's Degree, he married Brenda. He
credits his improved outlook resulting from his participation in
wheelchair sports for his success in courting Brenda. "Before then I
had always felt no woman would ever marry me."

Today, Bill is a happy man, far different in attitude and social
ability from the high school dropout of years before.

"Not long ago, I told my father I now thought that there had been
some good things about my becoming a paraplegic. He thought I
was crazy. The point I was trying to make to him was that being
paralyzed forced me to do some good things with my life that I probably never would have done otherwise."

Bill and Brenda have a close relationship with all the athletes in
New Life, but they have a special regard for Sylvester Fiers, who
has been with them the longest. Sylvester became a paraplegic at
the age of 15 months when his baby highchair fell on him. He met
Bill when he was 13, a skinny, unsure kid who desperately wanted to

29

engage in an organized sport. A student in the school where Bill was a counselor, Sylvester felt defeated because the wheelchair basketball team would not let him play. They felt he was too thin and, therefore, not strong enough to propel a chair fast enough to compete on the court. In addition, the school's sports adviser did not want Sylvester to use a wheelchair yet, advising that he use the braces and crutches as long as he could. Most physical therapists want paraplegics to remain upright on crutches as much as possible.

"Once youngsters who have been pulling themselves awkwardly and slowly around on braces and crutches get into a wheelchair, they fall in love with its speed, ease, and comparative grace," explains Bill, "and they don't want to get up on those slow crutches anymore."

The problem is that people who sit down all day long get a lot of infections in the urinary tract.

But despite the team's feelings about his lack of strength and the sports adviser's recommendation that he not use a wheelchair, Sylvester was determined to play baskeball. He just would not take no for an answer. He persisted in his quest, stubbornly cornering Bill time after time in his office. Impressed by the young pupil's determination, Bill eventually relented and made him a member of the *New Life* basketball team.

But he would remain on the team, Bill solemnly warned Sylvester, only as long as he spent all his time when he was not on the court, upright in his braces and crutches. Sylvester agreed to the condition.

It took Sylvester months to learn how to shoot baskets while sitting in a chair. At first he couldn't even hit the rim. But he worked so hard that today he is one of the top scorers for the *Capital Smokers*. In 1980, in addition to his Olympic medals, Sylvester won three events at the 24th National Wheelchair games in Illinois. He took first place in the 200, 400, and 800-meter dashes. Sylvester credits his success to the chair he borrowed for the events and had used for only one day. The importance of the chair was explained by Bill.

"See, we have the wings to fly around the court," he said laughing and flapping his arms, "but we just haven't the right equipment to let us show what we can do. We have been competing on chairs with 24-inch wheels, while everyone else was competing on 26-inch or 27-inch wheels. So our kids have been borrowing. They look around to see who has the fast chairs and borrow them."

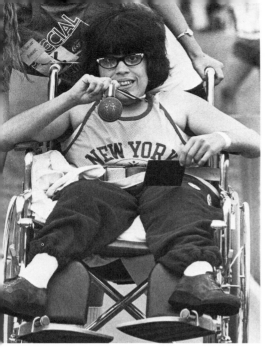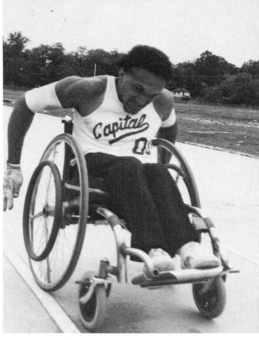

A wheelchair athlete shows off
her medal. *Courtesy Special
Olympics*

Eric Ramey, team member of
Capital Smokers, gets ready for
a practice session. *Photo courtesy Brenda Greene*

The specialized chairs for sports events have covered spokes. The
wheels are canted to lower the center of gravity. And they have better ball-bearings in the wheels so they roll faster and with less effort.

Bill is very aware that participation in organized sports teaches
handicapped people many things about the larger game of life. According to Bill, the wheelchair games instruct the players how to
cope with the inevitable give and take of daily existence.

"Handicapped kids are somewhat possessive and self-centered,"
he says. "I am teaching them to give more of themselves and to
learn to be less demanding of others. In sports, you have to be able
to lose gracefully, and I am teaching them that they can't have im-
mediate gratification for every one of their wishes. I am trying to
push kids to learn how to do things cooperatively, how to work with
people, and how to get things done, because those are vitally necessary life skills."

There are more than 140 wheelchair basketball teams across the
country. In addition to basketball, track and field events, and swimming, there are many other sports for wheelchair athletes—touch
football, softball, tennis, bowling, archery, and there is—would you
believe it—even square dancing.

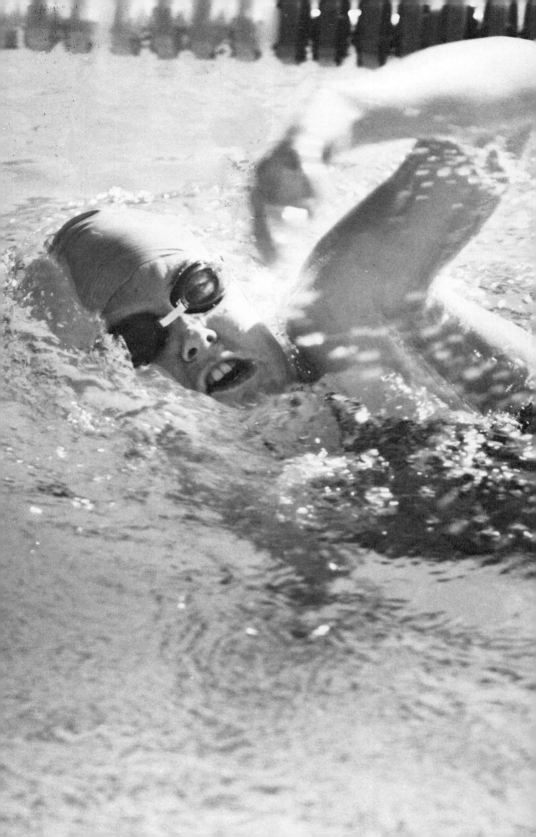

Swimming

At the 1980 Summer Olympics for the Disabled held in Arnhem, Holland, American athletes captured 73 medals, more than any other country.

Among the Americans, the swimmers were the top performers, bringing home 38 medals.

Among the swimmers, the most dazzling performer was 16-year-old Trischa Zorn, who is legally blind. She won a hard-to-believe total of seven gold medals and, in addition, set seven world records. She was judged to be far and away the outstanding athlete in the Olympics for the blind.

Trischa's goal is to compete in the 1984 Summer Olympics for the sighted in Los Angeles. "I want to show that handicapped people can do things that sighted people can do," she explained.

Trischa should not have any trouble achieving her goal. She already does most of her competitive swimming against sighted athletes and is a familiar figure at national swim meets around the country.

Her best event is the backstroke. One of her former coaches, John Mason, rates Trischa as one of the top 40 backstrokers in the nation.

At a recent North vs. South meet in California, Trischa placed second in the 200-yard backstroke. Her time of two minutes, six and 8/10 seconds qualified her for a spot at the National AAU championships in the Spring of 1981 held at Harvard University in Cambridge, Massachusetts. Trischa was off her best time by one second. Trischa's reaction to the dropoff in her first AAU meet? "Just wait till next year!"

A junior in high school, Trischa lives in Mission Viejo, California. She is 5'8" and weighs 120. She began swimming when she was eight.

Trischa Zorn swimming the Australian crawl during practice workout. *Photo courtesy Mission Viejo Company*

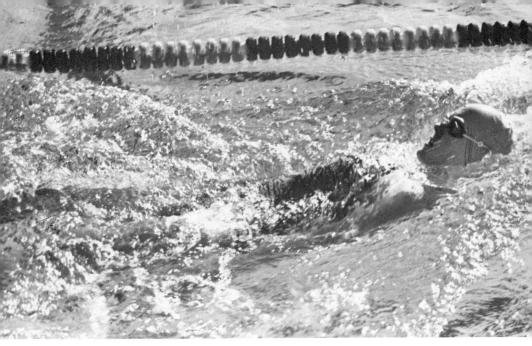

Trischa Zorn does the backstroke. *Courtesy Mission Viejo Company*

Trischa gives her mother, Donna, a lot of credit for her success. Her mother's sacrifices have been considerable. She drives Trischa to all of her meets and makes it possible for her daughter to keep up her rigorous training schedule. Every day, Donna and Trischa get up very early, so that Trischa can be at the Mission Viejo Nadadores Club pool to begin her workout at 5:30 a.m.

Trischa exercises 5-1/2 hours a day, two hours in the morning before school and two hours after school. In between, she lifts weights and runs about eight miles a day.

Trischa also acknowledges the hard work of her swim coaches, who have worked with her so unselfishly, she says. She has a great deal of pride in being a member of the Mission Viejo Nadadores Club, since it produced two former Olympic champions, Brian Goodell and Shirley Babashoff. Trischa wants to join their company.

In school, the young swimmer maintains almost an "A" average. Her excellent schoolwork and athletic ability have brought Trischa scholarship offers from some of the top colleges around the country. "I am being offered swimming scholarships, but I haven't made up my mind yet where I'll go," she said. "I want to study physical education for the handicapped."

During practice, swimmers use a pace clock to regulate the speed of their swimming. Trischa's teammates read the clock for her. She usually swims in lane number one because one edge of the lane is the well-marked pool wall, which makes it a little easier for a swimmer who has almost no vision to keep on course. She wears special goggles because she was born with a rare eye condition, *aniridia,* in which a person's eyes have no irises and are an open lens. Trischa says the goggles help her a little. "When I was younger and swimming backstroke, I couldn't see the flags, so I ran into the wall a lot. I never do that anymore."

"Almost never, anyway," her mother amended with a proud smile.

Trischa explained that she can tell how close to the end of the lane she is by the number of strokes she has taken. Donna basically agrees with her daughter on that point. "But," she said, "occasionally Trischa under-estimates how far she has travelled and runs into the wall. On the other hand, she has over-estimated how far she has swum and misses the wall completely when she turns. But that is pretty rare."

Her poor vision, Trischa said, doesn't mar her relationship with other members of her swim team. "It doesn't bother them. They

Trischa Zorn, blind swimmer with Mission Viejo Nadadores Club. *Photo courtesy Mission Viejo Company*

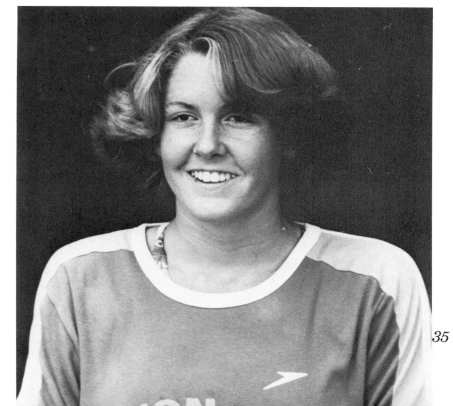

35

treat me as a regular and that is the way I want it."

With her heavy athletic schedule and squeezing in homework, Trischa has little time for teenage activities.

"You have to give up a lot as a competitive swimmer and I don't get to be with my friends as much as I'd like," she said.

"She'll probably make it to the 1984 Olympics," said her mother, "but to do it she's got to keep working, working, working. It doesn't leave her much time for a social life."

Not all disabled swimmers want to train for the Olympics. For others, swimming is simply the enjoyable time when they can take off their braces, get out of their wheelchairs, drop their crutches, and move with freedom. "For the disabled, water is as comfortable as crawling into a giant support-stocking," said Kathy Plant, a swimming coach for the handicapped. "A swimming pool is one of the few places they can enjoy the kinds of easy movements that almost everyone else takes for granted. Handicapped people don't walk funny in water, they don't look funny in water. When they submerge, the water pressure around them starts their circulation going."

Kathy recently became handicapped herself. She contracted multiple sclerosis, a disease which mysteriously hits young adults between the ages of 25 and 30. Now in her early thirties, Kathy explained, "MS is a disease which makes you feel fatigued. Frequently I will say to myself, 'Oh, no, there is no way that I can drag myself over to the pool and teach those disabled children.' But the kids just pull me out of it. It isn't the children, however, it is the water. It is the best place for me to be."

She has been teaching swimming to the handicapped since she was a teenager. "The nice thing for me is that I am giving these people a life skill, something they can do for the rest of their lives."

Kathy taught swimming for the District of Columbia's adaptive swimming program for special education youngsters. Through that program she met Bill and Brenda Greene of *New Life,* who asked her to train wheelchair athletes as competitive swimmers. She gladly took on the challenge. To make sure she was physically able to do the job, she repeated her Red Cross water safety instructor and advanced lifesaving tests.

(Top) Water is one of the few places the handicapped can move with freedom. *Courtesy The American Red Cross.* *(Middle)* A counselor communicates with a deaf child. *Courtesy The American Red Cross.* *(Bottom)* A blind swimmer holds the instructor's arm to learn the correct swimming motions. *Courtesy The American Red Cross*

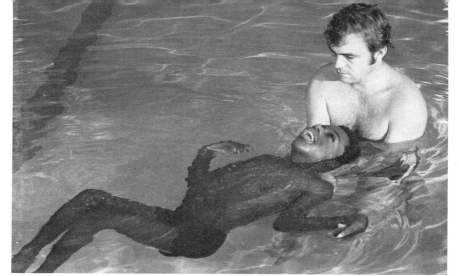

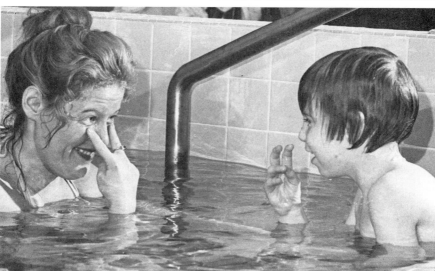

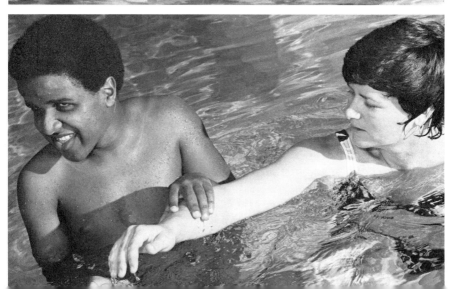

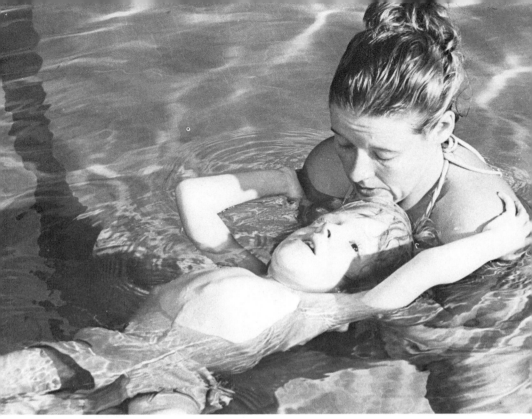

Getting a little help with the back float. *Courtesy The American Red Cross*

"I didn't need to, but I wanted to prove to myself that I wasn't a fraud. I wanted to prove I was able to save someone's life because frequently I would be the only competent swimmer in a pool area. I needed to know that even though I have a crippling disease I could do some quick, strong swimming.

"So I took a very tough course last summer. There were 16 students in the class. Only two passed the course and I was one of the two. I outswam the youngsters. It sounds as if I am bragging, but I was so surprised. I thought I would fail. But experience paid off for me. The bottom line is that once I hit the water, I am invigorated."

For Kathy, the swimming pool is a place where she can teach the handicapped, and a place which helps her own disability. "The physical contributions of swimming are important, but everyone should understand that your emotional well-being adds to your physical well-being," she explained. "Swimming is not a cure-all, but for the handicapped, it is a terrifically success-oriented activity. It combines the good feeling of being active and the good feeling of succeeding. So it helps your emotional well-being too."

Another expert on swimming for the handicapped agrees with Kathy. She is Louise Priest, who wrote *Adapted Aquatics,* the Red Cross textbook on teaching swimming for the handicapped.

"Several years ago, when I was teaching," said Louise, "a little kid got in the pool and he propped himself against the corner and said, 'You know something, Louise, this is the only place in the world where I can walk.'" Based not only on this eyewitness account, but on years of experience, Louise says water provides the disabled with the opportunity to do things they can't do anywhere else.

Carol Beaulieu, Aquatic Program Coordinator for Fairfax County Park Authority in Annandale, Virginia, goes one step further in

A member of the Bell System's volunteer organization, the Telephone Pioneers of America, helps a handicapped child into the water. *Courtesy The Pioneers of America*

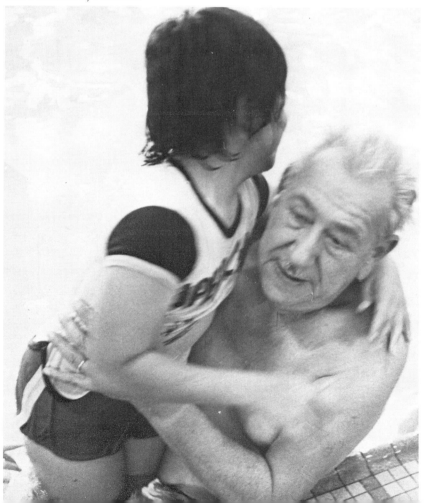

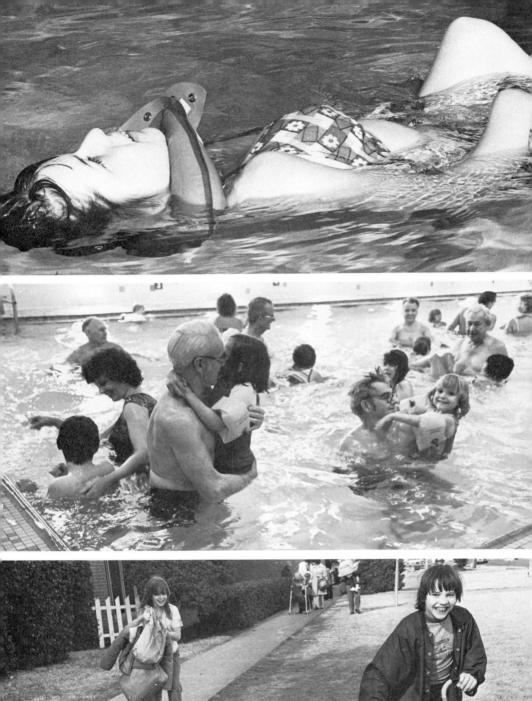
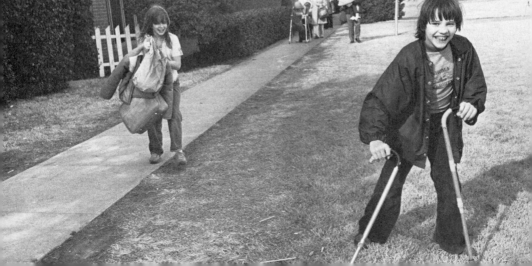

describing the beneficial qualities of water therapy for the handicapped. Carol says she knows handicapped children whose academic performance improved as a result of swimming. "Movement exploration and water games can be translated into school work very easily," she explained. "They learn in the water," for example, "how the body moves through space and they learn the meaning of words like 'in', 'out', 'around' and 'through.'"

Carol runs a year-round program that combines fun and games with instruction. Before disabled children are enrolled, she requires a physician's permission. She asks the cooperation of the physician in spelling out for her why they recommend swimming, what kinds of movements should be avoided, and what kinds of movements should be emphasized. The course of study for the disabled is structured around the doctor's recommendations. During school months, the children swim twice a week. During the summer, they swim every day. Carol and Louise say that at one time physicians did not recommend swimming for children with cystic fibrosis or asthma. Today, however, many physicians encourage children with these handicaps to get into the water.

Expert instructors say that a disabled person should begin swimming at an early age. In Fairfax County, Carol is teaching six-month-old disabled babies. "We try to mainstream them into our normal baby classes as soon as possible," she said. "It is important not only for the baby, but also for the parents. The parents of disabled children benefit by getting to know each other. This opportunity gives them the support they need and they can share experiences."

"Whether you are talking about a six-month-old with Down's Syndrome or a 16-year-old who has been in an automobile accident," Louise explained, "the sooner you can get them into an aquatic program, the sooner you will enhance their movement capabilities."

There are no scientific studies to document the advantages of water activities, according to these experts. "But time and time again, I have seen handicapped people improve their self-image, strength, and flexibility through swimming," said Louise.

(Top) Moving comfortably and easily through the water with the aid of an inflatable collar. Courtesy The American Red Cross. (Center) A group of Pioneers introducing handicapped children to the joy of water. Courtesy The Pioneers of America. (Bottom) A delighted handicapped youngster who participates in the Pioneer swim program. Courtesy The Pioneers of America

From her lengthy teaching experience with the handicapped, Carol has learned to be cautious about negative thinking. "The instructor must never set a limit," she said firmly. "I love to get a child about whom a doctor or some other expert has said, 'he never will be able to do this, or that,' even when in my own mind, I might agree with the diagnosis. For these children are fascinating to work with. Time after time—more frequently than I would dare to guess they could—they have surprised me and accomplished what we all thought was impossible for them. That is one reason I love this job. I get far more out of working with these children, I feel, than I can ever give to them. It's an exciting thing to do and it's work that's full of love."

While the majority of handicapped persons do not require any special equipment, some do, and only a few pools in the United States have been built to accommodate the disabled. The Fairfax County pools, for example, have ramps so that those in wheelchairs can wheel themselves into the water. They transfer from their own expensive wheelchairs into a cheaper water chair that can be rolled into the water without being ruined.

But even in pools that do not have built-in arrangements like ramps, there are many devices that have been adapted to help the disabled. And, if the device is not available, then in all likelihood someone will invent or improvise on the spot. One of the most inventive groups of people who work with the handicapped are the Bell System's *Pioneers*. Its members are mostly retired telephone workers and they are the world's largest voluntary association of industrial employees. A chapter can be found in almost every American and Canadian city. The *Pioneers* devote a great deal of time and effort to working with the handicapped. If a special bit of equipment is needed for a handicapped swimmer, a *Pioneer* will probably sit down and invent it or go out and find it. They have come up with such items as softballs and horseshoe games that beep, which enables blind children to play with them.

"Whenever you talk about aquatics for handicapped persons, you must always remember safety," Louise counsels. "I strongly advise that disabled persons be taken into the water only by trained personnel," she says. "They are available nationwide, primarily through the Red Cross and the Y's. They are excellent people and any disabled person who wants to learn aquatics should take advantage of their training and experience."

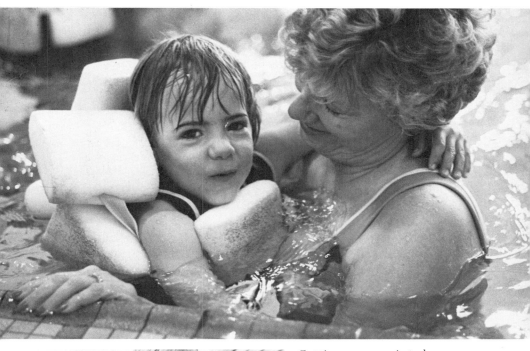

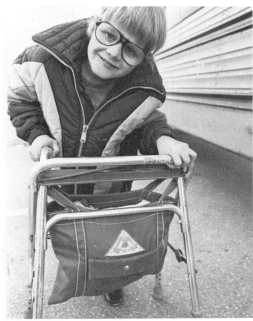

Getting acquainted with the water, aided by floats and a Pioneer. *Courtesy The Pioneers of America*

Dressed and ready for home after a Pioneer swim party. *Courtesy of The Pioneers of America*

43

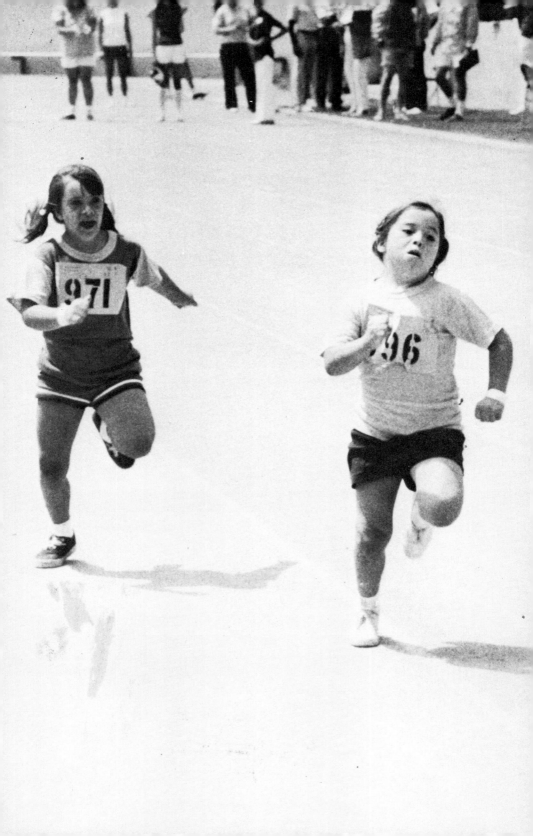

Track and Field

Harry Cordellos was born with glaucoma. While he was going through grade school and high school, he underwent eight operations and they partially restored his sight. But after he finished his schooling, his eyes began to fail again. In a desperate effort to save his partial vision, Harry's parents had him undergo six more operations. They failed. At age 20, after 14 operations, Harry Cordellos was totally blind.

In addition to failing eyesight, Harry had another major physical problem. He had what doctors call a heart murmer, a defect in his heart. His terribly concerned parents became over-protective of Harry. They wouldn't allow him to play games with other children.

"Because of my heart condition, I wasn't even allowed to play ring-around-the-rosy," Harry recalls.

That was bad enough, but he was to be punched hard by yet another devastating experience. While Harry was growing up, his father developed diabetes, which caused him to go blind. For the older man, losing his sight meant that life was all over for him. He became severely depressed and refused to enjoy life. He just sat around and would not let others help him to understand that there was no need to drop out, that he could still live a rich, full life.

His father's attitude was a terrible example for Harry. Like his father, he too just sat around the house. He turned into a sickly, frightened, depressed young man who spent most of his time listen-

Making a gallant effort to reach the finish line. *Courtesy Special Olympics*

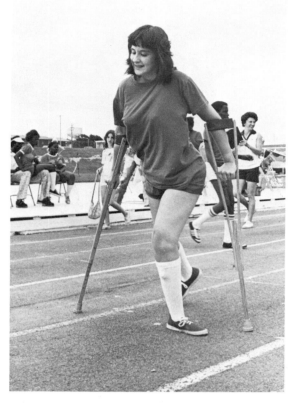

Nothing is going to stop her from reaching her goal. *Courtesy Special Olympics*

ing to soap operas and quiz shows on television, or else day-dreaming.

Then the doctors told Harry's mother that he had outgrown his heart condition. His heart was now all right and he could be physically active. She insisted he attend the Oakland Orientation Center for the Blind, which is near their home in San Francisco. There he learned to read Braille, to get around on his own by using the long cane, how to cook, and how to use power tools. They also taught him to improve himself physically through workouts in the gym. When they decided he had improved his stamina enough, an instructor took Harry to a nearby lake to teach him to water ski.

"He explained a little, but only a little, about water skiing," Harry recalls. "Then he put the skis and a life jacket on me. I was scared out of my mind, because I didn't know how to swim. But the instructor explained that the jacket would hold me up and that he would be watching every second. If I got into trouble, he would jump in the water right away to help me. He was emphasizing safety and his words helped, but I was still pretty scared.

"He handed me the rope handle and told me that when I was

ready, to yell 'hit it.' I did what he said and what happened in the next five minutes changed my life forever."

The experience was so important to him that more than 23 years later Harry remembers the exact day. It was August 17, 1958, and he was 20 years old. Learning that he could water ski—something he had never dreamed was possible for him—turned Harry into a different man. Since that day, he has never looked back.

He now has more self-esteem than he ever had while he was growing up and he has learned that there is practically nothing a sighted person can do that he cannot. Here is what he does now:

He water skis on two skis, on one ski, and on his bare feet. He skis on snow, both downhill and cross-country. He wind-surfs and goes hang gliding. He rides horseback and bicycles. He ice skates. He swims and has swum across wide San Francisco Bay, which has powerful currents that only strong swimmers can fight against. He is a high diver.

But of all his sports, Harry's favorite is long-distance running. Not jogging, but running of the toughest competitive kind in the world. Every year he runs about 2,000 miles and competes in 40 running events. He has run more than 50 marathons, which are 26-mile races.

Harry, who is now 43, has run several marathons in less than

Everyone's concentrating on hitting that tape. *Courtesy Special Olympics*

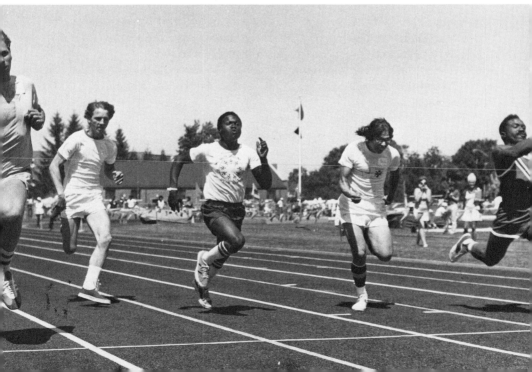

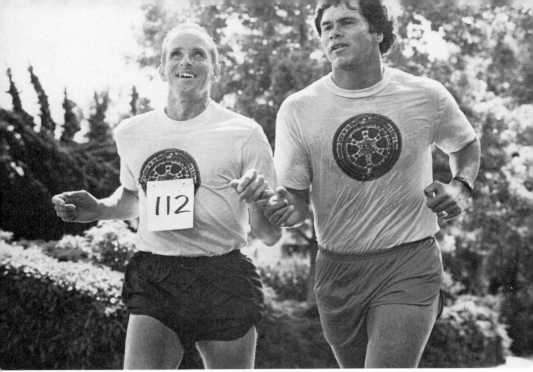

Harry Cordellos running with Jim Plunkett, Oakland Raider quarterback, whose parents are both blind. *Photo by Mark Tuschman*

three hours, which is a very good time, even for sighted runners. In 1975, he finished the famous Boston Marathon in under three hours.

The U.S. Marines sponsor a marathon every fall in the nation's capital. Harry ran it in November, 1980, and finished number 1,270 in a field of 6,800 runners. This achievement is all the more remarkable because only one month earlier Harry had undergone his 15th eye operation, in which his right eye was removed.

A month after his achievement in Washington, Harry ran the Honolulu Marathon, finishing about 500th in a field of 7,000 runners.

Harry runs with a sighted partner. At the start of a marathon, when the runners are bunched up and it is easy to run into someone, Harry lightly holds his partner's arm. After a few minutes, when the pack has spread out and the danger of collision has passed, Harry releases his partner's arm and they run with only their forearms lightly touching, their legs pounding in unison.

As they run, Harry's partner keeps up a steady stream of instructions and warnings to let Harry know what is ahead. As they approach a curve in the road, his partner will tell Harry, depending on which direction it turns, "inside curve ahead," or "outside curve ahead." As they enter the turn, his partner keeps repeating with each step, "curve, curve, curve," until they are through the turn. Marathons often include a trip up or down a stairway. As with a curve, his partner warns Harry that steps are coming up. Then as they reach them, for each step the partner calls out, "step, step, step." The same is done for sections of the route where projecting tree roots or stones make the going rough.

One of Harry's regular partners is Mike Restani, with whom he usually runs once a week. With Mike, Harry ran the Dipsea Course in California. This is a grueling seven-mile cross-country race which includes running up 300 steps, over a mountain covered with projecting roots and rocks, and down a steep ravine to finish near the sea. In a field of 2,000, Mike and Harry finished in the top third.

Mike says of his blind partner, "I never knew how intense Harry was about achieving in sports until I sat out a race and watched his face. He has an incredible drive, an intense desire to accomplish something, to show what he can do. His running proves that he can do better at many sports than most sighted people. Sighted or blind, it makes no difference, Harry ranks right up there with the best."

About what a blind person experiences while running long

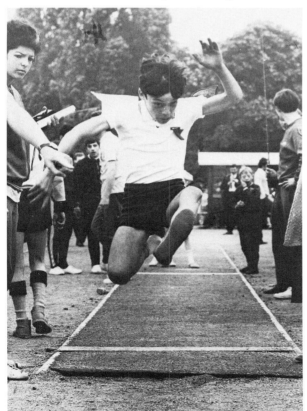

A runner in the making, practicing his jumps. *Courtesy Special Olympics*

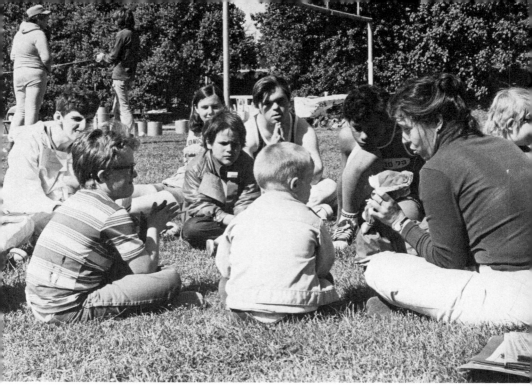

Young athletes being coached on the game's rules and regulations. *Courtesy Special Olympics*

distance races, Harry said this: "You might think it would be boring to run a marathon or to ski great distances cross country when you can't see what is around you. But it's not boring at all. I love outdoor sports because they bring me close to the beauty of nature. I don't see the beauty, of course, but I experience it in other ways."

In an interview with a California reporter, Harry described his impressions during a recent race, the Avenue of the Giants Marathon, 26 miles through the redwoods. "While I was running, I was just overwhelmed by the beauty of those trees, trees that I could never see. But I could smell them and hear the leaves in the branches rustling over my head, and feel the sounds of the runners' footsteps bouncing back off the big trunks. All that was wonderful. I mean, any blind person who says you can't appreciate to a certain degree your whole environment is just closing off the world."

For years, Harry has traveled all over the country, holding seminars and demonstration clinics to show both the blind and the sighted what sightless people can accomplish in sports. Wherever he speaks, he always stresses safety first.

"The big underlining I put under everything I tell audiences is that with every sport—no matter how daring or even how crazy it may seem for a blind person—it's never as dangerous or as crazy as it seems, like hang gliding, for instance, if everyone involved thinks safety first and always keeps it in mind. That's the key with everything for the blind, safety first."

Because of his willingness to do anything or go anywhere to help other disabled people, Harry recently was awarded a notable tribute. At the 1980 convention of the American Alliance for Health, Physical Education, and Recreation in Detroit, Harry was presented with the prestigious William Anderson Award. He was the second handicapped person to receive it.

To other sightless persons, Harry offers this: "All sports, but particularly running, have improved my confidence in my ability to do many things I used to think only sighted persons could do. Through trial and effort—lots of effort—I learned to overcome failure. You must never be afraid to try, and you must never be afraid of failing. To fail is not the worst thing in the world. After you have failed ten times, you will appreciate all the more the success that comes on the 11th try."

Harry's outlook is supported by Arthur Copeland, President of the U.S. Association for Blind Athletes. Founded in 1976, the ABA now has more than 3,000 members. The organization has enabled hundreds of blind athletes to do something they never dreamed they would be able to do—compete in high-level national and international sporting events. Mr. Copeland went on record recently, saying this:

"The only real problem blind people have is to be accepted and recognized as individual people who happen to be blind, and no dif-

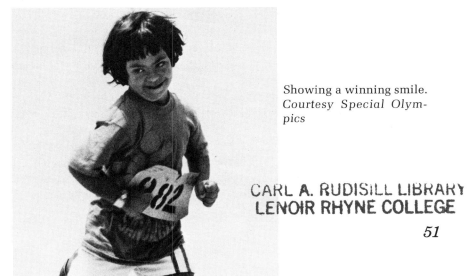

Showing a winning smile. *Courtesy Special Olympics*

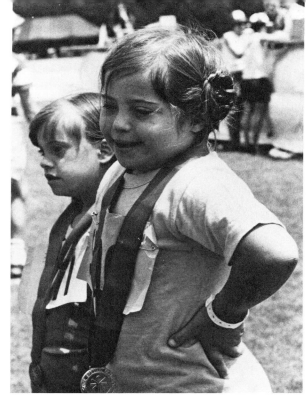

Two happy winners, enjoying the sunshine and cheering their friends. *Courtesy Special Olympics*

ferent from you and me. Our gospel is to recognize them as athletes and not as blind athletes."

For the parents of blind children, Harry has this strong, but practical advice:

"You must never assume that just because you are sighted, you have all the answers for your child. Your child is a person in his own right, just as much as you are. He has his own ways of learning and his own time for learning. You must never assume that because your blind child isn't able to learn something now that he will never be able to learn it. That's a terrible mistake and my parents and I are good examples of a family that made that mistake. Adaptive techniques that are rapidly being developed for blind people have made it possible for them to do things that no one would have believed possible for them 20 years ago."

Adaptive techniques made it possible for Harry to hold down a job as an information clerk for the Bay Area Rapid Transit System in San Francisco.

"Here I am, totally blind, telling sighted people how to get around this big and busy city," said Harry, with a booming laugh that

"Here I am, totally blind, telling sighted people how to get around this big and busy city," said Harry, with a booming laugh that showed how much he appreciated his accomplishment. "For me, being an information clerk is mostly a matter of having a telephone switchboard that was designed to use lights adapted for me with audio signals. I also transcribe train schedules into Braille and I have trained myself to remember a lot of facts about the system. It took time, but it wasn't too hard to do."

Harry threw back his head and laughed uproariously again. "I wonder what all those sighted people who have become lost in the system would think if they knew the guy who was giving them directions about how to get where they want to go was totally blind."

Asked how he could laugh about being blind, Harry replied:

"Because sports changed my attitude about myself. I like myself a lot better than I used to. Today I am a much happier person. I've learned to have faith in myself and to appreciate that while what I have isn't everything, it's a lot. I've learned to accept my lack of sight and to work within the confines of my disability rather than fight it and hate the world because of it.

"Besides, I think I've proved blindness isn't all that disabling."

Track and field champion Janet Rowley is frosted by a misconception she has found most sighted people have about disabled athletes.

"Sighted people believe that disabled people go into athletics only for therapeutic reasons," says Janet. "They tend to regard a blind athlete's accomplishments as significant only because they are therapeutic in nature. That's just not true and it has a tendency to put us down. We disabled athletes go in for athletics for exactly the same reasons as non-disabled people. We have fun in athletic compe-

A graceful high jumper makes it look easy. *Photo by Lil Junas*

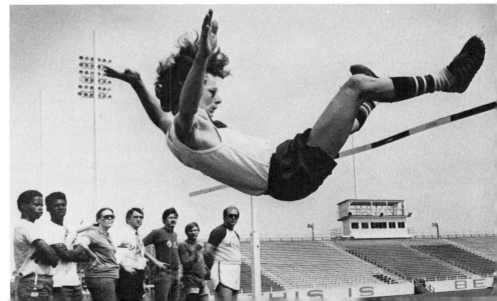

tition. We like having an outlet for our competitive instincts."

Janet got started in athletics at the Perkins School for the Blind, which is in Watertown, Massachusetts, near Boston.

"On my first day there, they took one look at me and told me I was going to be on the track team, that I was going to be a high jumper," recalls Janet. "They knew what they were talking about, I guess, because when they told me that I was 12 years old and I was six feet tall and skinny."

Janet is now 21, six feet three, 150 pounds, blonde, pretty and vivacious. She is in her senior year at Boston University, studying rehabilitation services for the handicapped. She is legally blind, with vision rated at 20/400. She can see only large shapes in a narrow range directly in front of her. When she goes into Boston alone she uses a cane to get around.

At the 1980 Summer Olympics for the Disabled in Holland, Janet threw the shotput 8 meters, 9 centimeters, which is an Olympic record for the blind. But she also holds the world's record from previous competitions of 9 meters, 45 centimeters. She also competed in the discus throw, the javelin and the pentathalon, which is a five-event series including shotput, running long jump, 100 meter dash, quarter-mile or 400 meter and 100 meter freestyle swim.

In the 1980 North American Games for the Handicapped, Janet set the new world's record for the shotput and the discus throw. She took first place in the high jump and in the pentathalon. She placed second in the triple jump and the long jump.

At the 1978 National Championships of the U.S. Association for Blind Athletes, Janet placed third in the long jump, second in the triple jump, and took first in the high jump with a distance of 5 feet and 1/4 inch.

At the annual competitions of the Eastern Athletic Association for the Blind, the trophy for outstanding athlete went to Janet for three years in a row.

The young athlete explained that if she were sighted and jumped five feet, it would not be a winning height, merely average.

"If I were able to make a running start like sighted athletes," she said, "I might be able to jump six feet, which would be very good. But who knows? I'm happy with my five-foot jump."

The high jump is her favorite event and also the one she is best at. She explained how she goes about getting over a bar she cannot see without knocking it down:

"I walk up to the bar and touch it and measure where it is in rela-

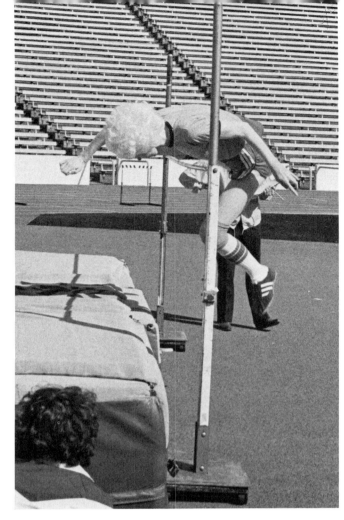

Janet Rowley clears the high jump at the 1979 National games in Seattle, Washington. *Photo by Norma Rowley*

tion to my height. That lets me know at exactly what height it is in relation to my body. I draw a mental picture of where it is. In every event, I use a lot of mental imagery, but the imagery is most important in the high jump.

"After touching the bar, I move back exactly three steps. We can take as many or as few steps as we want and I have found that three is the most comfortable for me. Sighted jumpers take a much longer running approach than we can, which is why they can jump higher.

"Three steps is not too far away from the bar for me. That distance gives me just the right amount of confidence. I know exactly how far away the bar is and how high it is. Once I have the distance and the height relationships all lined up in my mental image, I take the three steps pretty fast and just jump."

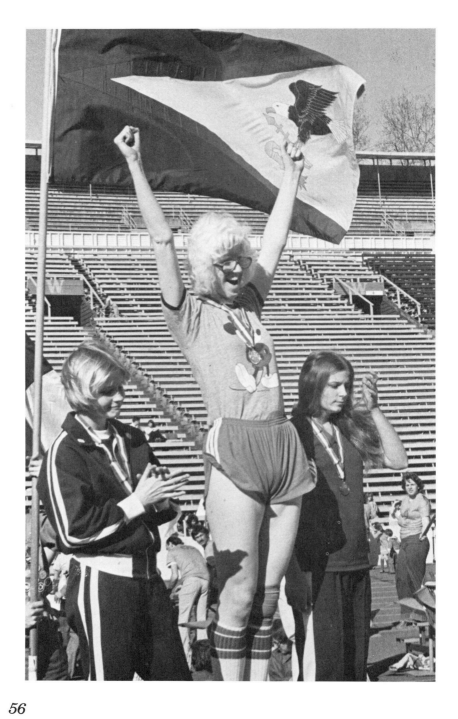

To train, Janet does the same things sighted jumpers do. She works out on a Universal gym and does calisthenics and stretching. When she is getting close to a competition, she trains three to four hours a day.

In addition to competitive sports, this talented young lady figure skates. She plays the piano, the organ, and the guitar. She square dances a lot. She has a good voice and is often asked to sing at weddings.

Like Harry Cordellos, Janet feels strongly that the attitude of a handicapped child's parents is probably the single most important element in whether the child will be a failure or achieve success in life.

"In most cases, the parents are not handicapped," she said, "and they just have no idea what their disabled child can or cannot do. They usually are too protective and they put barriers around their child that shouldn't be put there. They won't let their child do anything that has a little risk attached to it for fear the kid will hurt himself or herself. A lot of mothers, for instance, won't let a disabled girl do anything in the kitchen because of fear she will burn herself. Such overprotection hinders the child's development in later life.

"Parents have to realize that their child will have to be self-sufficient at one point or another. They should not restrict their children when they want to do something, especially around the house. A handicapped child might as well do things when their non-disabled siblings are doing them. Disabled children should be allowed to fall or get bumped or scraped sometimes so that they will learn for themselves what they can or cannot do. Knowledge of how far they can push themselves is invaluable and a bump or a scrape is a cheap price to pay."

Blind track and field star, Janet Rowley, cheers after receiving the first place medal for high jump. *Photo courtesy Norma Rowley*

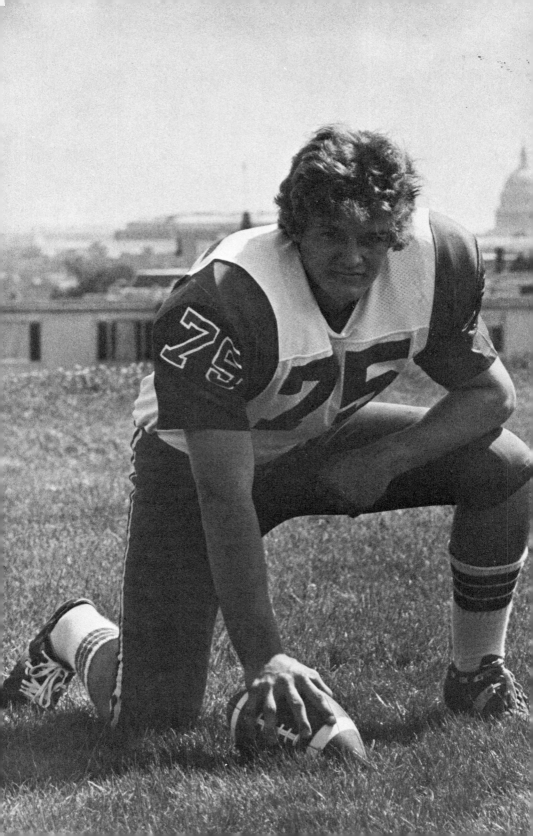

Football

Ron Symansky, the Eagles' 17-year-old defensive tackle—six foot four and 220 pounds of hard muscle—dropped into the set position and looked his opposing lineman right in the eye. The visiting team's center snapped the ball to his quarterback, who dropped back two steps, arm upraised to throw a pass. But he took just a second too long to spot his receiver. An Eagle got through the screen and sacked the quarterback hard. The ball flipped into the air. Ron, the graceful giant, leaped high and snagged it, making the fast retrieval look as easy as plucking an apple off a tree. He tucked the ball against his side, danced around the tacklers who reached for him, and streaked 58 yards into the end zone.

The crowd roared, the band played, and the Eagles went wild.

But the touchdown hero heard nothing. He is deaf. As Ron Symansky walked to the sidelines, he was happier than he had ever been. A smile split his face from ear to ear. "Even when I go to Heaven, I'll remember that day," he said recently.

When he was younger, Ron Symansky never dreamed he would one day be a football star. In his early teens, Ron was as skinny as a beanpole, awkward, and uncoordinated, because he did not know how to exercise. He was an easy target for some bullies in his Massapequa, New York, neighborhood, who thought it was fun to pick on a deaf kid. They often sent him home crying.

Ron Symanski, 1980 captain of the football team of the Model Secondary School for the Deaf. *Photo by Peter J. Moran*

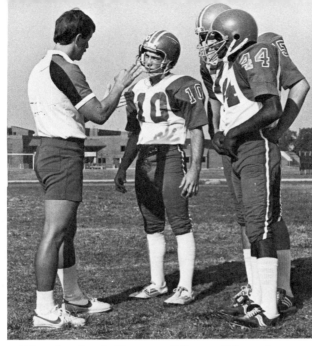

Coach Bob Westermann signing his instructions to MSSD Eagles. *Photo by Peter J. Moran*

"On the football team, I learned how to exercise and I gained weight and became tougher," Ron recalls. "Now those kids who used to beat me up hide when they see me coming."

Ron is captain of the Eagles and has been twice named to the All-Star team of the Maryland-Virginia Football League. "Football is so important to me," he says with a laugh, "that when I sleep, I dream football."

The Eagles are students at the Model Secondary School for the Deaf, which is on the campus of Gallaudet College in Washington, D.C. Gallaudet is the only liberal arts college for the deaf in the United States. It was established by an Act of Congress in 1863. The graduates of Gallaudet have the distinct honor of having the President of the United States sign their diplomas, a tradition that has been followed since the college opened. Ten years ago Gallaudet established the Model School for high school students as a demonstration project for other deaf secondary schools in the country.

Not until 1977 did the Model school decide it would be a good thing for its students to play football. To coach the team, they chose Bob Westermann, 29, who has a Master's Degree in adaptive physical education. People who earn this degree are specially trained to teach physical education and sports to those who are handicapped.

Bob began training four years ago with a bunch of raw recruits who barely knew how to handle the ball. Worse, coach and players had a big communication problem. Bob did not know how to sign.

60

But he learned fast because while he was teaching his players how to play football, they were teaching him how to sign.

Each season the Eagles play almost as many hearing teams as they do deaf teams. "Our first season, I thought I was very successful," coach Bob recalls. "We were three wins and five losses. When we started, we didn't have one boy on the team who knew how to snap the ball, quarterbacks had never taken an exchange before and they didn't know how to throw passes. Nobody knew how to block. And after only one training season, we beat three teams. That wasn't too bad, I figured, for a new coach who was learning sign language.

"But then something odd dawned on me: we had beaten the hearing teams. We had been zonked by the deaf teams. All things being equal, why should deaf teams that I knew weren't any better than us regularly beat us while we could beat pretty good hearing teams?"

For quite a while, Coach Westermann was baffled. He held many strategy sessions with his players, assistant coaches, and friends, but no one could come up with an answer.

Eventually, while they were watching the Eagles play another deaf team, several Model School teachers solved the problem. They saw the opposing team's coach using binoculars to read the instructions Coach Westermann was signing to his quarterback out on the field.

"I was just a rookie coach in the deaf league," Coach Westermann says with a slightly sad smile at the painful memory, "and those other coaches were taking advantage of me."

It doesn't happen any more because the coach no longer signs directly to the quarterback. Instead he delivers his instructions by messenger. And when he is signing the play to the messenger, the assistant coaches gather around them in a half-circle so that nobody on the other team can read Bob's message. The messenger then runs on to the field and signs the play to the team in their huddle, where the message is blocked from the view of the opposing players.

Football historians say the huddle was invented many years ago at Gallaudet College. In football's early days, the quarterbacks of hearing teams would shout out the play codes while his team just stood around on the line of scrimmage. Then they would line up and go. Deaf teams couldn't have their players just standing around any which way while the quarterback signed the plays, because one player might block another's view. So Gallaudet's deaf team came

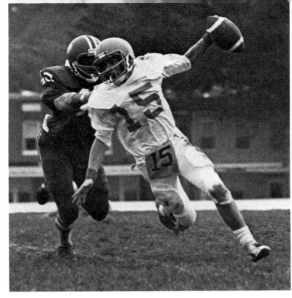

Wilfred Overby, MSSD Eagle (dark jersey), tackling Maryland School for the Deaf quarterback, Mike Baer. *Photo by Peter J. Moran*

up with the idea of having everyone move behind the line of scrimmage and bend over in a huddle so everyone would be sure to see what play the quarterback was signing. Hearing teams thought that looked like a pretty good idea and picked it up.

Both Coach Westermann and his players have learned fast and well together. The proof is in their remarkable record. In 1979, in only their third season, they captured the Deaf National Championship. And they did it again in 1980. The Eagles have steamrollered over both deaf and hearing teams without distinction. In their last seven games of the 1980 season, they were not scored against. During the entire nine-game season, only 16 points were scored against them. Also, in 1980, the Eagles flew to Miami, where they won the North-South Deaf Bowl Game against the Florida School for the Deaf.

Before joining the faculty of the Model School, Bob Westermann coached at a regular high school, so he has a solid foundation for comparing the strengths and weaknesses of deaf players and hearing players.

"One of the hardest tasks a football coach has while training a high school team is keeping up their spirit. The most important ingredients for a high school football team are emotional and mental dedication to the game. Our kids are special. No one can deny they are different from other kids. But that doesn't mean you have to set limits on their efforts to achieve physical excellence. They play with a lot of desire.

"I put them through a training program as tough as you'll find in any high school anywhere. By the time the season starts, these kids are really trained."

The training program includes a lot of running and a strenuous program of weightlifting. The coach also urges the members of the team to fill in the off-season time with basketball and wrestling so as to stay sharp. Football practice begins in late August.

One of the team's top players is offensive swing back and defensive corner back, Wilton Downs. He is fast and nimble and during the 1980 season, he rushed 740 yards. Wilton previously played football at another high school. Asked to compare the training program at that school with the one at Model School, he said: "During training with the other team I used to lose about 15 pounds in three weeks. With Coach Westermann, I lose 15 pounds in three days. He's really tough on us. But because of his tough training, we're in really top condition and feel great. And because of that, even when we play a hearing team, we don't feel handicapped at all."

Coach Westermann sees only one slight disadvantage for deaf teams when they play hearing teams. Reading the defense pattern before the ball is snapped, quarterbacks on hearing teams sometimes decide a switch in plays is called for and just shout out the new signal to their teams. When his players have their backs to him on the line of scrimmage, the quarterbacks of a deaf team cannot sign that he is going to switch to a different play from the one he gave the team in the huddle.

On the other hand, deaf players have an advantage over hearing players, according to the Eagles' coach. "I can remember Jesse Wade, one of my best players last year," he said. "I would give him

Wilton Downs, number 20, breaking away for a 78-yard touchdown run against Georgia School for the Deaf, an MSSD school record. *Photo by Peter J. Moran*

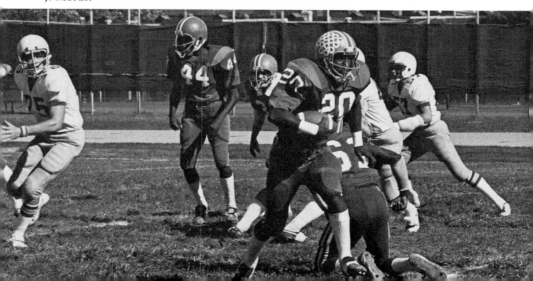

the ball 30 times in a game because he was so big and strong and such a good runner. He was such a thorn in the side of our opponents that when hearing kids tackled him, they would call him every name they could think of, trying to get his goat and throw him off his stride—forgetting, in the heat of the game, that he was deaf. But old Jesse just smiled at them because he didn't know what they were saying. He would just shrug and walk away. His relaxed response to their needling frustrated the hearing kids so much, I think it threw them off *their* game."

Another advantage for deaf teams seen by Coach Westermann is that deaf players very rarely incur offside penalties for moving before the ball is snapped. And that's because of something unexpected—on the line of scrimmage deaf players depend on *sound* to tell them when a play is starting. The sound comes from a drum on the sidelines. It is on wheels, and it is big—more than three feet in diameter. One side of the drum has been removed, which turns it into a sound cannon that shoots out powerful vibrations. As the team gets into position, the drum is wheeled along the sidelines to the line of scrimmage. When the drummer beats it, the drum shoots out powerful sound waves and the deaf players can feel the vibrations. In the huddle, the quarterback signs to the team whether they should go on the first, second, or third beat of the drum. Not having the distractions that come from hearing the cheering of the crowd and other noises, Coach Westermann believes, allows his players to concentrate on feeling the drumbeat and it is their concentration that causes them to have very few offside penalties.

Deaf players have no problem understanding referees' penalty calls since the refs use signs to tell spectators what has happened.

"Our parents understand very well how important it is for their boys to be successful at athletics," explains Coach Westermann. "Success—that's the key to their whole psychological development. When they succeed, it lets them know they *can* do things like other people. They have the tremendously important experience of discovering that if they really work hard at something, they have ability to succeed at it. After that experience—no matter how often they get put down during their lives—they will know: If I work hard at something, I can succeed at it. It doesn't matter that I can't hear.

"For deaf kids, playing football has a far more important effect than just teaching them they can succeed at something physical. It has a profound psychological effect. Succeeding at an organized team sport helps end the isolation of deaf people from others."

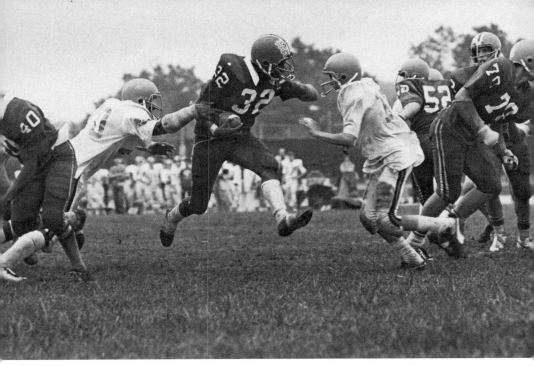

Jesse Wade, number 32, running for a touchdown against Maryland School for the Deaf, assisted by blocking of Ron Symanski, number 70, at right. *Photo by Peter J. Moran*

Wilton Downs confirmed the coach's observation. "Before I played sports, I didn't know many people. But after I joined the team, a lot of people wanted to know me and I made a lot of friends. People seem to look up to football players more than they do with players of other sports."

Being on the team has even brought Wilton closer to his five brothers and one sister, all of whom have hearing and who felt he was different from them. Before he joined the team, they had always kept themselves a little apart from him. But then he succeeded at the game; his name often appeared in the newspapers and his mother started a scrapbook. One day, one of his brothers told Wilton: "Hey, Wilton, you're just like the rest of us now. Welcome to the Downs family!"

Wilton Downs may be on the brink of the greatest achievement yet for a deaf player, which is to be able to play on a hearing team. He is now being approached by a college. Wilton has slight hearing, which can be boosted with a hearing aid. This, together with his ability at lip reading, permits him to follow a conversation between hearing people.

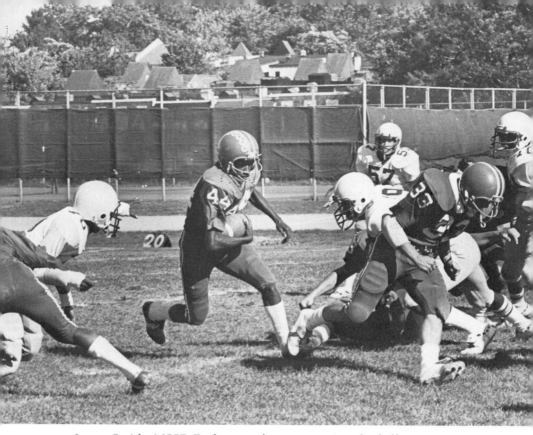

James Smith, MSSD Eagles, number 44, running the ball against Georgia School for the Deaf. *Photo by Peter J. Moran*

Football changed Ron Symansky from a timid, awkward boy, so badly coordinated that he easily lost his balance. Today he is a self-assured, superb athlete. Ron is preparing for college with the goal of becoming a football coach for the deaf. He wants to follow closely in Bob Westermann's shoes.

"The deaf can do just about everything in sports," says Coach Westermann, "although there are a few games in which they must contend with communications barriers. In basketball, for instance, the players talk to each other constantly. The deaf have a harder time in basketball because they need eye contact to communicate. In races and sprints they are at a slight disadvantage because when they are in the blocks they have to look up so they can see the smoke come out of the gun. The hearing runner's head will be down, which is more advantageous. With a few limitations like this, the deaf definitely can play everything. But I think they play football best.

"I think our kids play with a tremendous amount of desire and drive because they want to prove to those who can hear that they are nothing less. Deaf people meet a lot of frustration. Adolescents might go to a store to buy something, for example, and maybe the sales people don't want to spend the time with them to communicate. The deaf meet these frustrations day in and day out. The football field is important because it is one place where the deaf can prove themselves. They can say, in effect, to those who can hear: 'You're not better than I am. I am your equal. In fact, I might even be able to beat you!'"

Ron Symansky agrees with his coach on that: "When we play a hearing team they think because we're deaf we can't play. But we've proven them wrong—many times over."

For the Eagles' coach, his most enjoyable moment comes when he sees the happiness of the players after they have beaten a hearing team. The Eagles take off their helmets, walk across the field, and shake hands with the losers. "And all the time," says Bob Westermann, "the grins across their faces are saying, 'We did it! We did it!'"

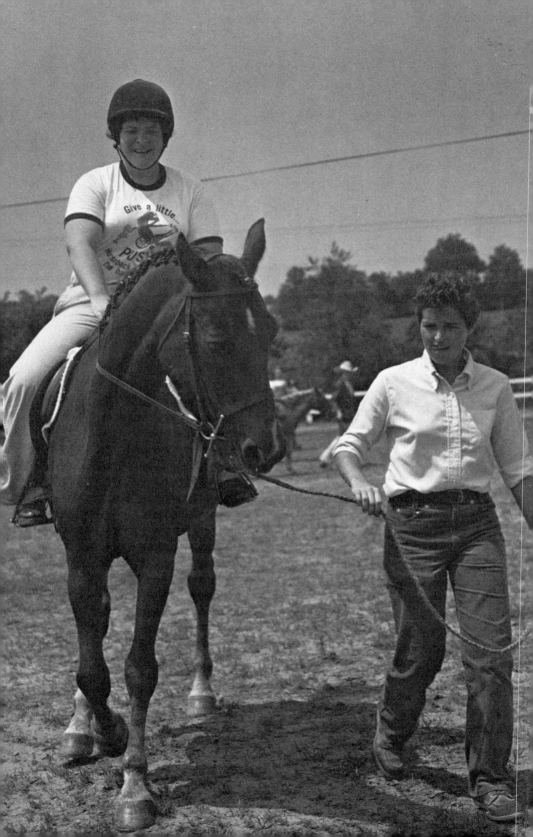

Horseback Riding

A new sport for the handicapped got started in the United States about 15 years ago. Unlike most of the other sports in which handicapped people engage, this one is definitely intended to be therapeutic. It produces some amazing results for children and adults with a wide variety of disabilities.

It is horseback riding.

But that's only an expensive hobby for well-to-do people who have lots of time—and are normal—isn't it?

Not any more, it isn't.

Wendy Shugol, 31, who has cerebral palsy, is a rider skilled enough to be picked to ride for the U.S. in international competition in 1980. This is what she said riding has done for her:

"For one thing, it gives me a tremendous psychological lift, because it is nearly the only sport I can participate in where I am absolutely free. I have four good legs under me and I can keep up with any able-bodied person who happens to be riding with me. On the ground, I'm always lagging behind and asking people to wait up for me. But on a horse, I can go just as fast as any able-bodied person or even pull ahead of them. Wow! I might even be a better rider than they are and be able to go faster than they can. And that's another wow!

"But just as important—*more* important even—is what riding does for me physically. I can walk only with braces and it is quite painful because the muscles on the inside of my thighs have tightened up so much that my hip joints no longer fit properly in the sockets. When I am seated on a horse, my thigh muscles are stretched and my hip joints move into their correct seating and it relieves my pain.

Wendy Shugol on her favorite mount, led by Georgeanne Alexander, coach, National Cerebral Palsy Games.

"I start my riding sessions with my muscles and entire body rigid. I cannot even get my feet into the stirrups. But as I take my horse through his paces, adjusting my body movements to the rhythm of his movements and the heat from his body soaks into my muscles, I begin to relax and loosen up. Pretty soon my legs get relaxed to the point where my feet can be placed in the stirrups. It always amazes me to feel this happening to my tightened and rigid muscles.

"More than two years ago my doctor began saying I would have to have drastic surgery on my hips. But the riding has been so good for me that he has kept putting off the surgery. And not long ago he put it off again—for a whole year this time. I felt like going out to the barn and kissing my horse!"

After a ride, Wendy gets some carryover. For a time on the ground her walking and balance are much improved.

Why does this happen? Nobody knows for sure. Some research is now going on to try to find out what in the brain is released to cause the improvements on horseback that is not released when the rider is on the ground.

Her experience gained in five years of riding has led Wendy to suspect this:

"A lot happens to a person on horseback. A person has to readjust his body constantly when he's in the saddle. Every time the horse moves, the rider has to do something, sometimes consciously, sometimes unconsciously. This goes on all the time and there's an awful lot of kinesthetic and tactile exchange between the rider and the horse. The rider's joints get a lot of new input and new sensations."

Wendy's riding is backed up by physical therapy sessions three times a week to relax her thigh muscles. So impressed was the therapist with what sitting on a horse was doing for those muscles that he built her "Clyde"—a wooden horse that stands in her living room. When she is at home, Wendy's riding saddle is cinched on to Clyde and she sits in it while watching TV or reading. The effect is similar to riding a live horse, keeping her thigh muscles stretched and relieving her pain by permitting her hip sockets to fit into place.

Wendy was not disabled until she was 22. Not long after graduating from college with a degree in adaptive physical education she fell and struck her head a hard blow. The resulting hemorrhage caused brain damage and cerebral palsy. Now both legs and both arms are affected and she walks with leg braces and Canadian crutches. She has lost the ability to crawl on her hands and knees, to

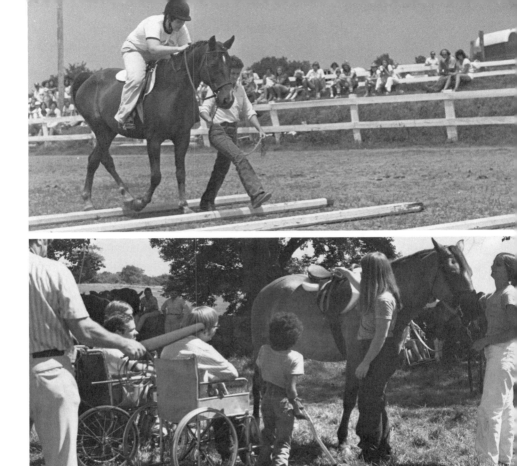

(Above) Wendy Shugol at Loudon 4-H Fair on "Marquee" lead by Coach Georgeann Alexander. *Photo courtesy Wendy Shugol.* *(Below)* Riding students receiving a lesson on tack. *Photo by Duffy*

roll over, or to kneel unsupported. She no longer has her protective reflexes, so when she loses her balance her hands and arms do not react to try and break the fall. Despite these problems, Wendy insists on walking as much as she can. In the school where she works, however, she finds the distances too great for her and she has to surrender to a wheelchair. She is a teacher of physical education to disabled children in Fairfax, Virginia.

The first handicapped person in the world who undertook a therapeutic riding program was an Englishwoman named Liz Hartel. She was a great rider, but in the late 1940's she contracted polio. Her doctors told her that because of her disability she could no longer ride. Against medical advice, she and her family started riding

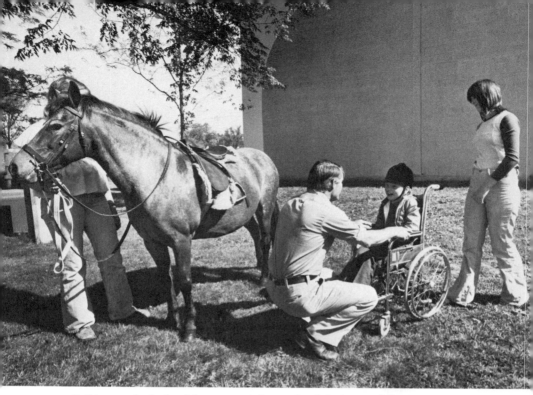

Getting ready for her big moment, from wheelchair to saddle. *Photo courtesy North American Riding for the Handicapped Association*

again. The therapeutic effects worked so well that she went on to win a silver medal in the 1952 Olympics—the Olympics for normal people, that is.

This great success for a disabled rider caused some physicians in Europe to do some research, which led to the present training programs. The idea took many years to reach the United States.

Wendy believes so keenly in the benefits of therapeutic riding that she has become a spokeswoman for the sport. She is frequently invited to lecture on it throughout the country. Her aim is to help handicapped children, to recruit volunteers, and to raise donations for the volunteer riding program that taught her.

Wendy learned to ride in the Riding for the Handicapped Program of the 4-H Club in Loudon County, Virginia. The program operates six days a week, each spring, summer, and fall. It does not operate during the winter because the disabled riders are affected strongly by cold. Each year, 85 children are taught to ride. The club owns ten specially trained horses.

The Loudon 4-H Club is part of the North American Riding for the Handicapped Association (NARHA). It is an all-volunteer, non-profit organization in the United States and Canada. Leonard Warner, Executive Director, has volunteered ten years to the program. There are 140 NARHA centers in 37 states and Canada that serve about 4,000 disabled persons each year. The organization has at least as many volunteers who teach and assist with the program. Financial support comes from donations by individuals, school systems, corporations, and foundations. There is no charge to students. All of NARHA's affiliated programs must fulfill tough standards, practice stringent safety precautions, and give their volunteer instructors rigorous training.

President of NARHA is John Davies, a former British Army cavalry instructor. In Chidwell, England, he founded one of the earliest programs for teaching the handicapped to ride. A few years ago he moved to the U.S. and now works with the Cheff Center in Augusta, Michigan, which is the largest program in the nation for teaching riding to the handicapped. Cheff is where most NARHA riding instructors have been trained.

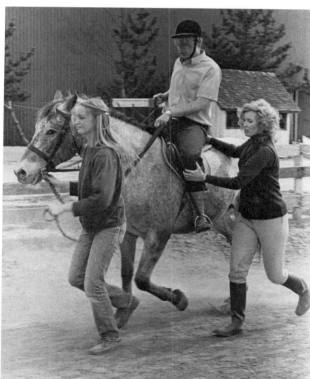

Kenneth Streicher aided by Joan Athen. Vicki Horton leads the horse. *Photograph courtesy Maryland Therapeutic Horsemanship Association*

One of them is Joan Athen, who was trained by John Davies. Joan now runs a riding program in Columbia, Maryland, and in it, she explained, she stresses safety first.

"We have safety equipment for people with all different types of handicap. With most of our trainees, in the beginning we have a side-walker on each side of the horse and a third walker who leads it. The rider doesn't even have to have balance, for we have belts with handles on them and the side-walkers can hold the rider upright until he learns to hold his balance on the animal. This is the way we do with new people week after week while they get used to sitting on a live animal and learn to balance on it."

Joan said there was almost no physical handicap she could think of that would prevent a person from learning to ride to at least some degree. Her program has equipment that will permit even people with pronated hands, that are locked into a closed fist, to hold and pull the reins. They have reins with wooden hoops on the end that they place on the rider's arms so they can pull the reins. If they cannot use their arms to pull the rein, they are taught to turn their body from side to side when they want the horse to turn. The animal has been trained to respond to the change in pressure and will turn as the rider indicates. So even people who can't feed themselves, who can in fact, do nothing for themselves, can turn a horse under them.

Neither is age much of a barrier. Joan sets a lower limit of age five, but she has no upper limit. Her oldest student to date was a woman aged 60.

Joan stressed that all trainees in NARHA programs must have their doctor's permission to participate and the program must have a full medical description from the physician of the trainee's disability. Where the person has a physical therapist, the therapist must also understand the riding program and cooperate with it.

Of the program's therapeutic elements, Joan said this:

"To the trainees, we don't stress the therapeutic element. They come to us to have fun and their goal is to learn to ride. And they do learn. But while they are doing so, we do many other things for them that they are not aware of. For instance, often when a child first gets on a horse for his lesson, he won't be able to lower his legs below the level of the animal's mane. In a matter of minutes, the horse works his miracle. Its movements and its warmth begin to work and soon the youngster can lower his feet and place them in the stirrups. That's the therapeutic part.

"Another part of the therapy is the emotional lift a disabled child

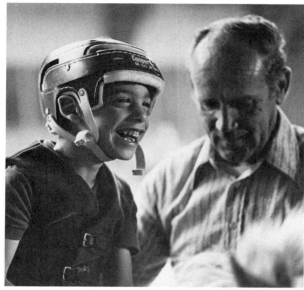

59

Safety headgear for this young rider while astride his pony. *Photograph by the North American Riding for the Handicapped Association*

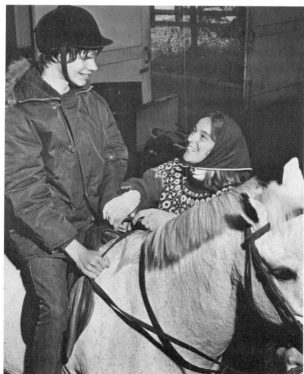

60

Jerome Fisher, 14, is reassured by instructor Jean Mc-Cally. *Photo by William L. Klender*

gets from riding. For the first time they are doing something that many normal people cannot do. The ability to ride makes the handicapped person unusual. Handicapped people are nearly always underdogs, the ones who can't do what normal people do. But riding is something about which they can say to a normal friend who doesn't ride: 'This is something I can do that you can't do.' For the handicapped child that knowledge has incalculable value."

Joan explained that one of the peculiarities of being on a warmblooded animal is that the experience makes the autistic child more mentally alert, while it causes the hyperactive child to calm down.

"Actually, I can get autistic children to ride by themselves without assistance faster than children with any other handicap. When I have an autistic child on a horse and he seems to be totally out of it, I will suddenly clap my hands and it snaps them back to right now! Today! Now! They look at the horse and say, 'Oh, my gosh! It's just me and this horse and if I don't do something right now this horse is going to run away with me.' They will act and react and work harder than anyone else because they realize it is just them and that horse—against the rest of the world. They get that kind of relationship with the horse and realize they have to do things for themselves."

Another part of the therapy is the empathy that develops between rider and mount. The children become quite affectionate toward the animals. They soon settle on one mount and demand to ride it at every session.

One of Joan's trainees was 12-year-old Emily Shearn. At every riding session she demanded to ride "her" pony, which was named Vicky. Before she started riding, Emily was confined to a wheelchair. After getting to know her pony, she named the chair Vicky. Emily graduated from the chair to braces and a stroller after she learned to ride. She promptly named the stroller Vicky.

Emily's mother, Peggy, described her daughter's progress as a result of riding.

"The riding was good for her, especially for trunk control. She now needs fewer people to help her. The rhythmic movements of the horse relax Emily and she needs that. Once on the horse, she has a freedom of movement that she cannot get in any other way and that's tremendously important for her self-esteem.

Joan Athen instructs Emily Shearn on "Vicky." *Photo by Joe B. Mann*

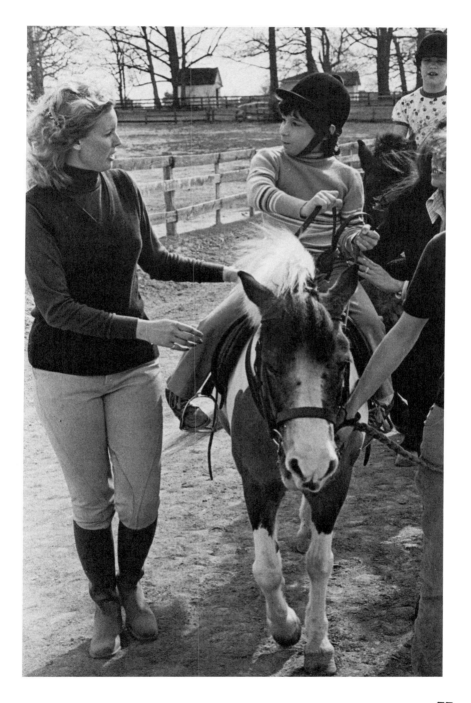

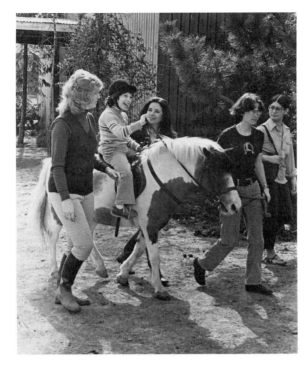

Emily Shearn rides "Vicky." Joan Athen, left, and M.T. Gutmanis, on the other side of Emily. *Photo courtesy Maryland Therapeutic Horsemanship Association*

"Another important thing for Emily is being able to control that huge creature and make it do what she wants. Emily can control nothing else in her life, not even her own body, and here she has this animal following her commands.

"Riding has given her great self-confidence. When riding, she never has a qualm. She just gets up on the horse and tells it to go. She never has an anxious moment. The power she has learned she has over this animal, that she has nothing to fear from him, has given her great self-confidence and great self-esteem. Those are valid feelings for her that she never had before.

"Not to mention the fun and the joy that goes along with all this."

Resource and Sports Organizations Serving the Handicapped

American Alliance for Health, Physical Education, Recreation and Dance
1900 Association Drive
Reston, Virginia 22091
(An information center providing educational materials and films on handicapped athletic programs)

American Athletic Association of the Deaf, Inc.
3916 Lantern Drive
Silver Spring, Md. 20902
(Promotes state, regional, national and international basketball, softball and volleyball tournaments each year.)

American Blind Bowling Association
150 North Bellaire Avenue
Louisville, Kentucky 40206

American National Red Cross
17th and D Streets, N. W.
Washington, D.C. 20006
(Special swimming programs are offered for the handicapped in many cities. Call your local chapter for information.)

American Wheelchair Bowling Association
224 North Federal Highway
Apt. 109
Boynton Beach, Florida 33435

Blind Outdoor Leisure Development, Inc. (BOLD)
533 East Main Street
Aspen, Colorado 81611
(Provides volunteer services to the blind who want to ski, ice skate and participate in winter and summer sports.)

Boy Scouts of America
Scouting for the Handicapped Division
Route 1
North Brunswick, New Jersey 08902

Camp Fire Girls
Handicapped Division
450 Avenue of the Americas
New York, N.Y. 10011

Council for National Cooperation in Aquatics
9765 Bragg Lane
Manassas, Virginia 22110

The Exceptional Parent
Statler Office Building
20 Providence Street
Boston, Mass. 02116
(Bimonthly magazine carries articles on many sports topics for parents of disabled children and teenagers.)

Fairfax County Park Authority
4030 Hummer Road
Annandale, Virginia 22003
(Aquatic program for the handicapped.)

Federal Aviation Administration
Department of Transportation
Washington, D.C. 20591
(Provides information about flying for disabled pilots, as well as the portable hand controls which can be installed in general aviation aircraft for paraplegic pilots.)

International Committee of the Silent Sports
Gallaudet College
Florida Avenue and 7th Street, N.E.
Washington, D.C. 20002
(Winter and summer sports programs for the deaf. Also write to Model Secondary School for the Deaf at same address for more information on football for the deaf.)

Kids on the Block
Suite 510
The Washington Building
Washington, D.C. 20005
(Put out a newsletter entitled, "Keeping up with the Kids," which has useful information for parents with handicapped children.)

Maryland Therapeutic Horsemanship Association
P.O. Box 1031
Columbia, Maryland 21044

National Amputee Golf Association
24 Lakeview Terrace
Watchung, New Jersey 07060

National Foundation for Happy
  Horsemanship for the Handicapped
Box 462
Malvern, Pennsylvania

National Foundation for Wheelchair
  Tennis
3855 Birch Street
Newport Beach, California 92660

National Park Service
Department of the Interior
18th and C Streets, N.W.
Washington, D.C. 20240
(Information on camping and recreational facilities accessible to the handicapped.)

National Spinal Cord Injury
  Foundation
369 Elliott Street
Newton Upper Falls, Massachusetts
  02146
(For information on the Boston Marathon)

National Wheelchair Athletic
  Association
Nassau Community College
Garden City, New York 11530
(Information on wheelchair track and
  field sports.)

National Wheelchair Basketball
  Association
University of Kentucky
110 Seaton Building
Lexington, Kentucky

National Wheelchair Softball
  Association
Box 737
Sioux Falls, South Dakota 57101

New England Handicapped
  Sportsmen's Association
P.O. Box 2150
Boston, Mass. 02106
(Summer and winter sports for the
  handicapped.)

New Life, Inc.
Capital Wheelchair Athletic
  Association
2300 Good Hope Road, S.E.
Washington, D.C. 20020
(Competitive wheelchair basketball,
  swimming, track and field events)

North American Riding for the
  Handicapped Association
Box 100
Ashburn, Virginia 22011
(Serves as an advisory body to nation-

wide chapters in therapeutic and recreational riding for the handicapped.)

Special Olympics, Inc.
1701 K Street, N.W.
Washington, D.C. 20006
(Nationwide organization for recreational and therapeutic sports program for
  mentally retarded.)

Sports 'n Spokes
5201 North 19th Avenue
Phoenix, Arizona 85015
(Bimonthly magazine for wheelchair
  sports and recreation.)

Sportsline
University of Illinois
117 Freer Gymnasium
Urbana, Illinois 61801
(This university is considered the mecca
  of wheelchair sports. They publish a
  newsletter six times a year on sports
  information for the handicapped.)

United Cerebral Palsy Association, Inc.
66 East 34th Street
New York, N.Y. 10016
(Wide-ranging sports program for
  victims of cerebral palsy.)

United States Association for Blind
  Athletes
55 West California Avenue
Beach Haven Park, New Jersey 08008
(Nationwide sports program for blind
  athletes to compete in national and international events.)

U.S. Blind Golfers Association
6338 Sherwood Road
Philadelphia, Pa. 19151

U.S. Olympic Committee
Handicapped in Sports Committee
1750 East Boulder Street
Colorado Springs, Colo. 80909
(To provide the prestigious support of
  the American Olympic Committee to
  handicapped athletes who participate
  in competitive sports program.)

U.S. Deaf Skiers Association
159 Davis Avenue
Hackensack, New Jersey 07601

Wheelchair Motorcycle Association
101 Torrey Street
Brockton, Mass. 02401

Wheelchair Pilots Association
11018 102nd Avenue North
Largo, Florida 33540

Winter Park Recreational Association
Box 36
Winter Park, Colorado 80482
(Provides ski instruction to handi-
  capped regardless of disability; also
  have a summer sports program.)

SPORTS
FOR THE
HANDICAPPED

By ANNE ALLEN

Opportunities exist today that were undreamed of only a few years ago for disabled individuals to participate in active competitive sports. This inspiring book tells of and illustrates some of the recreational activities and sports available to handicapped persons—aquatics, basketball, football, track and field events, skiing, horseback riding. Besides capsule stories about individual athletes, it lists addresses for organizations and programs throughout the United States that are devoted to sports for the handicapped. Illustrated with photographs.